SLEEP
The Secret of Problem-free Nights

Beatrice Hollyer
and
Lucy Smith

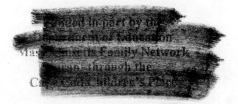
Funded in part by the
Department of Education
Massachusetts Family Network
through the
Cape Cod Children's Place

WARD LOCK

For my mother
B.H.

For Robin and Emma
L.S.

A WARD LOCK BOOK

First published in the UK 1996
by Ward Lock
Wellington House
125 Strand
LONDON
WC2R 0BB

A Cassell Imprint

Distributed in the United States
by Sterling Publishing Co., Inc.
387 Park Avenue South, New York, NY 10016–8810

A British Library Cataloguing in Publication Data block for this book
may be obtained from the British Library

ISBN 0 7063 7504 1
Typeset by York House Typographic Ltd
Printed and bound in Great Britain by Biddles Ltd

Cover picture: *Collections/Sandra Lousada*

CONTENTS

Funded in part by the
Department of Education
Massachusetts Family Network
grant through the
Cape Cod Children's Place

FOREWORD

IF I HAD just one ambition when I brought my new baby home, it was that she would sleep. Lack of sleep makes my head feel as though it is full of cotton wool, and I had a feeling that I would need my wits about me. And I wanted to do more than just survive. I wanted to enjoy my baby, and help her enjoy her new life. I was going to need energy, and that meant sleep.

New babies are notorious destroyers of sleep. You can spot their parents by their dazed expressions, and the characteristic thousand-yard stare from sleep-starved eyes. I was already horribly familiar with this fierce survival instinct towards sleep from my years as a breakfast television presenter, when my alarm went off at a brutal 3am and my afternoons passed in a blur worse than jet lag.

I didn't want life with a baby to be like that. I knew what I did want: adult time in the evenings, a chance to have a break from the baby and recharge my batteries. And I wanted to sleep all night, so as to leap from my bed refreshed and eager to greet the dawn – but preferably not before 7am. Of course that's what I wanted. Doesn't everybody? But how do you get it? And is it even possible? My mother was sceptical. 'You can't *make* a baby sleep,' she would offer as dubious comfort over supper in the first weeks, while the baby looked up winsomely from her car-seat carrier under the table. Luckily for me, by then I knew Lucy.

Lucy first came to our house as our health visitor, when my daughter was ten days old. Like a fairy godmother, she made my wish for a soundly sleeping baby come true. She showed me that, although of course you can't *make* a baby sleep, you can help him. You can teach him; you can show him how it's done, so that he is able and willing to do it for himself.

That's the theory – and it worked. When my daughter was a

month old, she began sleeping a 'core night' (one of the keys to this approach). Following Lucy's advice, I seized on this as a sign of her readiness to sleep all night. Well before she was three months old, her night lasted the magic twelve hours I had dreamed of – from 7pm to 7am. That pattern has survived all temporary disruptions. At eighteen months she plays in her cot on waking and never calls for attention before 8 or even 9 am.

She was not born a good sleeper. As a new baby she was wakeful, difficult to feed and in need of constant comfort and reassurance. In no way was she one of those blessedly peaceful infants who seem to doze the first couple of months away. That made me all the more convinced that what we both needed was sleep.

I read a lot of books, but it was always Lucy who made sense of it all. How do you establish bedtime at the time you want? Should the baby be left alone if she protests at bedtime, or should I stay with her? Or should I leave, but keep going back to reassure her? What if that just upsets her more? What should I do if she wakes in the night? Pick her up? Feed her? Leave her alone?

Not only did Lucy know the answer to these and countless other questions, but she also showed me why certain methods help and others don't. Fifteen years of hands-on experience with babies has given her a practical knowledge and understanding of what they need, and how they show it, that goes beyond anything I've read. I began to pass on Lucy's advice to friends struggling with wakeful babies. Even second-hand on the telephone, her methods worked wonders – once with a baby of a year old who had never slept through the night. If Lucy could make such a tremendous difference, I thought, everyone should have access to her methods. New parents often have to muddle through by trial and error. Although advice comes at you from all sides, and there is certainly no shortage of books, it can all be a bit bewildering – especially when none of it seems to apply to the way your baby is behaving at the time. You need the kind of knowledge that creates confidence and lets you respond to your baby in the way that's best for him. I had everything to learn, and to be guided by someone who really knew the territory was a blessing.

Although Lucy's approach does provide immediate answers to specific problems, the real difference is that it's a complete picture of what sleep means to your baby – sleep from your baby's point of view. It shows you how to help your own particular baby develop good sleep habits. It is sleep tailor-made for you and your baby, not a one-size-fits-all approach that fits nobody properly.

Every time I thought: 'Help! What now?', Lucy steered me back to first principles and reminded me how to read and respond to my baby's signals. Then everything settled down again, with me congratulating myself on my new-found parenting skills.

If anyone can turn a bewildered, anxious new mother into the smug, rested parent of a soundly sleeping baby, it is Lucy. This book unpicks her approach, to allow you to put it together again in the way that suits you. It gives you her methods, as well as the tools to adapt them to your own baby, and to your own preferences and circumstances. It makes you the expert on your own baby. That's the secret of problem-free nights. Finally, our deep appreciation and thanks are due to those parents whose thoughtful conversations about their babies inspired this book, to Dilys Daws of the Tavistock Clinic, whose book *Through the Night* (Free Association Books) brilliantly illuminates many of the mysteries of infant sleep, and especially to the countless parents and babies who shared their troubles and triumphs with Lucy over her fifteen years as a health professional specializing in babies and young children. Their experiences are the foundation of this approach to sleep. This book could not have been written without them.

Beatrice Hollyer
London, 1996

NOTE The problem of whether to refer to your baby as a boy or a girl is solved by alternation chapter by chapter. Therefore 'your baby' in the Foreword is a boy, but in the Introduction she's a girl, and so on. It's no more satisfactory than any other method, but it seemed the simplest approach. And except where mothers and fathers are specifically mentioned, everything is intended for either parent, or both.

INTRODUCTION

SLEEP is far and away the most commonly reported problem in babies under a year old. One clinical estimate suggests more than a third of babies of this age have sleep problems, and research shows that half of all babies who have a sleep problem at one year still have it at three. That little phrase, 'sleep problems', represents an enormous daily ration of stress, conflict, frustration, confusion, anger and sheer exhaustion for the parents and babies caught up in them.

Nobody wants a sleep problem. When you are expecting a baby, it's usual to dread the broken nights to come. After admiring your new baby, the first thing many people ask is: 'Does she sleep?'. Being deprived of sleep, especially over a long period, is a special kind of torture. But many people believe it's a matter of luck whether you are landed with a baby who sleeps well or one who doesn't. It isn't.

Of course, babies do vary enormously, in their sleep needs as in everything else. A placid baby won't need as much help in settling into good sleep habits as a jumpy one. But even babies who are born good sleepers sometimes become bad ones later on. And early sleeping through the night is no guarantee that your baby won't develop a sleep problem at some stage.

The truth is that whether or not your baby learns to sleep well is up to you. Your baby can't choose to sleep well or badly. But you can choose to make it easy for her. You can give her everything she needs, while still sending her the clear message that night-time is for sleep. While she is tiny, she is extremely receptive to your signals. If you show her how, reinforce her own steps in that direction and put no obstacles in her path, she will sleep well.

A baby who has been guided into good sleep habits from the beginning need never develop a sleep problem in the first place.

• Treating a Sleep Problem •

Of course, sleep problems, once they have developed, can be treated. This book shows how to identify what is causing your baby to be wakeful, so you can tackle the root of the problem. A head-on confrontation over sleep produces nothing but conflict. Understanding the reasons for wakefulness, on the other hand, builds trust and good communication between you and your baby, and allows her to relax and feel good about sleep.

Although it is primarily aimed at preventing sleep problems, and for that reason we focus on establishing good sleep habits from the start of life, this book can be used to solve a sleep problem in a child of any age. The principles are exactly the same. Applied to an existing sleep problem, they will allow you to get to the bottom of it and sort it out in a very short time usually less than a week. But this will involve making a few changes. As creatures of habit, babies and young children typically resist any change to their familiar routine. Extreme protests, though, seldom last more than a day or two. By the fourth or fifth night, your child is likely to accept the change and sleep through the night. Bear in mind that, for a couple of nights afterwards, she will very probably wake again. This is not a setback. She is just testing the new rules and she needs to find out that they're still in place.

It is much, much easier never to develop a sleep problem in the first place than it is to solve a problem once it has developed. A new baby's needs are very simple; a one-year-old's sleep problem can be quite complicated. For this reason the earlier you start encouraging good sleep habits, the easier things will be for all of you.

• HOW NEVER TO HAVE A SLEEP • PROBLEM

Good sleep habits start in the womb. That's because you hold the key to your baby's successful adaptation to sleeping all night. By the time she is born, you can be well prepared to help her, starting from day one. Easy, pleasant sleep, under her own control, is one of the greatest gifts you can give her. Foundations laid in infancy will stand her in good stead throughout her life, as she will always be able to draw on her early experience of bed as a peaceful place where her energies can be restored.

For you, of course, the rewards are more immediate. Your baby will settle into sleeping all night as soon as she is bio-logically ready to do so – and that may be much sooner than you thought. Even the liveliest baby will show the beginnings of it after just a month or so. Most healthy, full-term babies can sleep for twelve hours a night by three months. By six months, they all can. If it doesn't happen, something is preventing it.

Your baby is born programmed to adapt to sleeping all night. But this programme is easily thrown off course or delayed. Sometimes a baby is well loved and cared for, but the way this is done has the unwanted side effect of disturbing the natural process of adaptation and making her unable to sleep. On the other hand, by understanding her needs, watching her signals and following her lead, you can strongly reinforce your baby's tendency to adapt to sleeping all night, and it will happen quickly and easily as a result.

This approach to helping your baby sleep rests on three central ideas:

- The 'core night' is your baby's early signal that she is ready to sleep for long stretches at night. If you are on the lookout for this turning point, you can seize the opportunity it presents to consolidate your baby's sleep quickly into a whole, unbroken night.

- Babies don't sleep well by luck or accident. Sleep is a learned skill, and you can help your baby learn it from the first days of life.

● Without meaning to, you may make it impossible for your baby to sleep well. There are many different ways this can happen, ranging from how your baby goes to sleep, to feeding habits, to attitudes and feelings of your own. These can have a marked effect on your baby, even when you are unaware of them yourself.

Ideally, Chapter 1 should be read in pregnancy. There is no better time to begin thinking about your baby's sleep and to prepare to help her from the start. But knowing what sleep means to your baby, how sleep works and what we can learn from our own sleep needs are good first steps to helping your baby sleep, whenever you happen to read about them.

• WHAT ABOUT YOU? •

Chapters 2 and 3 are crucial to this approach. They are more about parents than babies, and there's a good reason for that. With the best will in the world, you can't succeed in helping your baby sleep if there's a confusion in your relationship with her that's sending her the wrong signals about sleep. Chapter 2 suggests ways of looking after yourself that will benefit your baby, and her sleep in particular. Chapter 3 shows how easy it is to prevent your baby from sleeping even while doing your best to help her, and how these pitfalls can be avoided.

These aspects of your baby's sleep are generally overlooked. Even when parents seek advice on sleep, they are seldom helped to discover the real reasons for their baby's wakefulness. So you end up treating the symptoms without knowing the cause, and if your baby's sleep does settle down, unresolved problems will often come back and disrupt it again. What's so cruel about this is that neither you nor your baby knows what's going on. You may be at your wits' end, having tried everything to help your baby sleep, and nothing has worked. These chapters help you to find the underlying causes of many sleep disturbances.

• FIRST STEPS TO SLEEP •

Chapter 4 looks at the first days and weeks of life, a time which, it's commonly believed, you can do little but survive. This is not true. The ways you find to settle your baby in her early days have a real influence on how she adapts to sleeping all night. Communication with your baby, which makes sleep and everything else run more smoothly, can also be established in the first days of the baby's life.

Chapter 5 contains one of the keys to this approach, the core night. This is the heart of your baby's own inbuilt sleep programme. If this signal is missed, her progress towards sleeping all night may be arrested and even reversed.

• FOOD AND OTHER HABITS •

Chapter 6 deals with the vexed question of food and sleep. Because they are so tightly connected at first, habits can become established that make it impossible to separate them and allow your baby to sleep all night. We look at how it happens that feeding is the most common cause of night waking in babies under a year old.

Chapter 7 describes sleep as a habit, and shows how closely it is linked to other habits and routines. These can be used to create positive associations and a relaxed state that makes it easy for your baby to go to bed and to sleep.

• WHAT TO DO WHEN YOUR BABY IS • WAKEFUL

However early your baby sleeps through the night, and however easily she does it, there will be times when, as part of her normal growth and development, she will have a wakeful patch. This is not a sleep problem, just a temporary hurdle for you and your baby to overcome. Chapter 8 shows how to make sure that a sleep problem never develops out of one of these episodes.

Chapter 9 discusses examples of special situations that can make you feel your baby can't be expected to sleep well, or make it hard to help her. Techniques for helping healthy babies to sleep are just as effective with ill babies, or babies with difficulties. We show how to apply these methods so that your baby sleeps as well as possible and her sleep continues to improve.

• TWELVE GOLDEN RULES •

Chapter 10 comes right back to basics. Once you have the knowledge you need to understand the influences on your baby's sleep, and how to manage them, the magic of this approach is its simplicity. It is summed up in twelve golden rules. Together, they are a trouble-shooting guide that will let you nip sleep problems in the bud. The rules are also a kind of map, to guide you reliably back on to the path of a good night's sleep, both for you and for your baby.

• BABIES AND BEYOND •

If your baby has learned good sleep habits in the first year of life, and you know how to steer her back on track when a disruption occurs, you need never have a sleep problem. The earlier you start, the easier it is. After a year she is likely to be set in her ways and to put up fierce resistance to changes she would have accepted happily when younger. A sleep problem, in a toddler, can be a deep-seated and complicated web of habits, opinions and will-power that can be difficult to unpick.

This book concentrates on babies up to a year old. However, it will still be of use to you if your child is older. To sort out any sleep problem, the first step is always to go back to basics. That means identifying the cause of your child's wakefulness and helping her sort it out, while still sending the clear message that night-time is for sleep. For a small baby, the message is wrapped in lots of gentle reassurance. A toddler is less easy to convince. But the goal is exactly the same.

Although the focus of this book is on babies, the principles can be successfully applied at any age. There is one exception: the golden rule, 'Never wake a sleeping baby', is no longer true when your baby becomes a toddler. By this age, a late-afternoon nap will interfere with her readiness to sleep at bedtime, so she may have to be gently roused at a certain time from her daily nap, and woken if she drops off at other times.

Nightmares, too, are more common in older children than in babies, and so are not discussed here in detail. But nightmares are just a more developed form of expressing anxiety, and the method for handling them is the same as whenever anxiety wakes your baby: reassurance, the minimum of fuss and disturbance, and a gentle but firm encouragement to return to sleep.

There is evidence that independent and self-reliant babies tend to be better sleepers than others. But good sleep feeds on itself. Learning to go to sleep by herself is a great leap forward in your baby's development, and encourages her dawning self-confidence and independence. In itself, a good night's sleep makes her more capable and good-humoured, so that she is better able to manage herself throughout the day. Then she goes to bed feeling pleased with her accomplishments and ready to relax. It's a positive cycle that starts with learning to sleep.

As for parents, you have only so much energy available. If your baby has trouble sleeping, it can drain your reserves with no end in sight – except, perhaps, the knowledge that by the time they go to school, most children sleep well. But five years of poor sleep is more than anyone should have to bear – especially parents of young children, who have plenty of other reasons to be tired. Instead of being wasted on just coping, your energy could be directed into a real achievement: a child who has always slept well and probably always will.

1

SLEEP BEFORE BIRTH
Pregnancy

'When I was pregnant, I slept badly. I suppose I just always thought sleep would be a problem for the baby, too.'

Mother of Gabriel, eleven months, who does not sleep through the night.

B Y ITS NATURE, sleep is hard to get a handle on. We need it, but we can't control it. Being a bit mystified by sleep ourselves can make it very hard to manage a baby's sleep. You may feel you can't plan for your new baby's sleep, as you plan for his feeding, changing and bathing. But you can.

• INFORMATION IN PREGNANCY •

People expecting a new baby are a captive market for manufacturers of baby food and equipment. Eager for information, determined to do their best for their baby, prospective parents are more receptive to advertising than most. Advertisers know this only too well.

But there are no profits in sleep. In our consumer society, this means no focus on sleep and no encouragement to plan for it. Sleep is not presented as something we need to consider and make informed choices about. That tends to be reserved for things we can buy. We are encouraged to channel all the natural uncertainties of pregnancy into shopping, and many unborn babies do become the eye of a hurricane of consumerism. But try to calm down, stop and ask yourself: What does a new baby really need? Milk, love, protection and sleep. And what do new parents crave? Sleep.

• THINKING ABOUT SLEEP •

When I was pregnant, my mother gave me a hand-woven cane basket and made it a lining patterned with stars. In my daydreams I imagined my baby sleeping peacefully in this basket. And so she did, the day she came home, for five blissful hours. And never again, for a whole month. She needed the reassurance and comfort of our arms. But I kept trying, and suddenly, one day, she was ready to sleep in her basket.

If I had given some thought to sleep when I was pregnant, I would have understood what was going on. I would have been less anxious for my baby to sleep, and she would have been able to settle down sooner as a result. Luckily for me, I began to learn Lucy's way of handling sleep when my baby was ten days old. But to learn it in pregnancy would have been better.

Pregnancy is the best possible time to start taking sleep seriously. It is very difficult to encourage your baby to sleep all night if you don't do it yourself, and perhaps have doubts that it is even possible. You can't just decide to sleep well, of course, and the discomforts and anxieties of pregnancy naturally lead to some bad nights. But what is important is to *believe* in sleep; to have clearly in mind the goal of a good night's rest for you and for your baby.

Once through the adjustment period, your baby may well sleep better than you do. One sleepless night I realized that my baby had been asleep for seven solid hours, while I hadn't had a wink. Her peaceful example encouraged me finally to get to sleep. But at first, when your baby is so much less of a separate person, it works the other way around. Your baby needs your guidance to learn to sleep well.

• HOW TO BE A GOOD SLEEP • EXAMPLE

You can use the time you are expecting your baby to start thinking about sleep and how it works. Even if you yourself are a good sleeper, this is a good idea, so that you will be able to help your baby learn what comes naturally to you.

Pregnancy inevitably means some broken nights. These wakeful moments are a good time for some sleep thoughts. How do we get back to sleep when we wake in the night? We need to be comfortable. We sometimes add a blanket, or throw one off. We need to feel sure that we are safe and that everything in our surroundings is normal. (Perhaps this deep-seated survival instinct explains why we sometimes prowl around the house before we can settle down again to sleep.) We need to clear anxieties from our mind and relax before we can let ourselves fall into unconsciousness.

Your discoveries about what helps you relax and sleep can be applied to your baby from the first days of his life. He too needs to be comfortable, at just the right temperature, relaxed and, above all, feeling safe and secure before he can allow himself to let go and sleep.

• FAMILY INFLUENCE •

There are such things as families of bad sleepers. That doesn't mean that a tendency to sleep badly is genetically inherited, but members of a family are likely to develop similar attitudes or habits around sleep. Parents of a wakeful baby often have a history of sleep problems themselves, like the mother quoted at the beginning of this chapter.

These attitudes are usually unconscious, so that parents are unaware of passing on to their baby their feelings that sleep is a difficult business. The best way to avoid 'programming' your baby to sleep badly is to recognize these habits of thought and behaviour of your own. Then it is possible to separate your problems with sleep from your baby's need to develop good sleep patterns. You will avoid getting locked into a family sleep problem, where your sleep difficulties are passed on to your baby and reinforced in turn by his wakeful behaviour.

If you send your baby the message that sleep is a good thing, easy and pleasant and safe, he will receive it, however unlikely this seems at first. If that idea is part of his first impressions of the world, it will become his own attitude to sleep and one of the automatic assumptions he will carry into adult life in his turn.

• ADAPTING TO THE WORLD •

Your unborn baby is accustomed to an uninterrupted drip-feed of food and to an environment with a constantly ideal temperature, muffled sounds and unchanging scenery. One day, your baby knows only the familiar security of the womb; the next, he is physically separate from his mother, feeling strange textures next to his skin and changing impressions from the air itself. Food is administered at intervals of several hours, creating the new and urgent sensation of hunger. The change is so great that it is surprising that your baby gets over the shock as soon as he does.

Babies, in fact, adapt to babyhood faster than we adapt to parenthood. That is why it is so often first babies that parents remember as difficult to 'settle'. By number two or three, you have got the hang of it. Your new baby picks up your confidence and is reassured, and that allows him to relax and sleep. But there's no reason why that reassurance shouldn't also be given to a first baby. Naturally you won't have the automatic ease that comes with experience. But your conviction and loving authority feel the same to your baby, whether you came by them through experience or not. You can decide what messages you want to send your baby and make sure you send them – without also sending a lot of others that contradict them.

• WHAT SLEEP MEANS TO YOUR • BABY

Sleep is a mental need as much as a physical one. It lets the muscles rest, but it is also the time when the experiences of the day are processed and integrated by the mind. This is doubly true for babies and children. Everything depends on how well they sleep.

They grow while they sleep, when the body can concentrate on building muscle and bone instead of expending energy. They wake after a sound night's sleep with a hearty appetite, having eaten or drunk nothing for as long as fifteen hours. That means the other big issue of infancy, food, goes smoothly as well: it is very satisfying to feed a properly hungry baby.

Above all, their brains sort themselves out while they sleep. A baby's day is an overwhelming deluge of new experiences and stimuli. So much is happening to him for the first time: first rain shower, first cold day, first hot one; first day barefoot on the grass, first fire, first dog.

Your baby has an urgent need for 'down time', when all this information can be mulled over and connected up with everything else. This ability to make connections is part of what we call intelligence. It is how your baby makes his experiences his own, so that he can draw on them and use them in the next situation he comes across. And sleep is when it happens.

• HOW DOES SLEEP WORK? •

We know that all night we alternate between cycles of deep sleep and lighter sleep. Deep sleep is the most restful and restorative. Dreaming stops, and mind and body relax fully. Lighter sleep corresponds with dreaming sleep, called REM sleep from the rapid eye movement that can be detected in this phase. REM sleep uses up quite a lot of oxygen and energy. You move around and may even speak.

It is only when we have the ideal balance of deep sleep and dreaming sleep that we feel well rested and refreshed by our night's sleep. We have all had the experience of sleeping all night, only to wake up still tired. This often happens when we are anxious, upset or depressed. It seems that mental stress keeps the mind busy, working through problems by dreaming, so we are deprived of more restful sleep at the deeper levels.

These two levels of sleep, deep or non-REM sleep, and dreaming or REM sleep, are both evident in babies in the last two months of pregnancy. Your unborn baby practises his breathing mechanisms during REM sleep, and the brain receives stimulation that helps the development of its higher, 'thinking' functions. Perhaps for this reason, small babies have more REM (or dreaming) sleep than do older children and adults. A baby will sleep very deeply after he first drops off, then stir and possibly wake after an hour or so. This cycle is repeated over the second hour. After that a baby may wake several times during a phase of dreaming sleep before he settles into another phase of deep sleep. He may wake several times more during the night as he switches between cycles of deep and dreaming sleep.

• WAKING IN THE NIGHT •

All these half-wakings can be seen as opportunities for an episode of being fully awake, if conditions are not ideal for continued sleep. When your baby wakes and cries, it means that his sleep cycle has reached a natural 'surfacing' phase and something is preventing him from going back to sleep. If he is sleeping well, he will just stir slightly, perhaps make a sound or two, then go back to sleep on his own.

Our own, adult, sleep cycles are similar, although the intervals between the repetition of each cycle are longer. We wake several times during the night too, although often we will not remember waking. We check on our surroundings, and perhaps change our position, before going back to sleep. This explains why we often sleep less well in a strange place. When we stir and half-wake, we get the message that our surroundings are not 'right', and that rouses us to full alertness. Of course, it is much more difficult to go back to sleep once something has caused you to wake completely.

This is the reason for one of the keys to this approach. If you put your baby to bed relaxed but awake, and let him fall asleep there on his own, when he half-wakes in the night, everything around him will be the same as it was when he went to sleep. His instinctive check sends back the message that all is well and that it is safe to go back to sleep. He need only repeat the process of falling asleep with which he began the night, and his parents are none the wiser.

If, however, your baby has been fed, rocked or walked until he is fast asleep, and then put to bed without rousing, when he half-wakes, everything will feel wrong. Where is the comforting nipple that was in his mouth? Where are his parent's protective arms? Checking on his surroundings will send back an emergency alarm signal, his instincts will go into a state of red alert, and he will wake fully and cry for help.

So we see that all babies, children and indeed adults, wake several times during the night, and babies even more frequently than older people. The only difference between a baby who sleeps well and one who wakes his parents with his cries is that a baby with good sleep habits is able to go back to sleep by himself after an arousal, while the wakeful one is not.

It often happens that parents establish a good bedtime routine, and their baby goes to sleep easily – only to wake and demand attention several times a night, or wake impossibly early and refuse to go back to sleep. This is one of the most frustrating things to deal with, because you feel, having got the baby contentedly to bed and to sleep, that there is nothing more you can do for him. But something is preventing him from sleeping well, and you will be able to find out what it is and sort out the problem, as we will see in later chapters. For now, though, it is important to understand that you will be showing your baby not just how to *go* to sleep, but also how to *stay* asleep – that is, go back to sleep on his own after a natural arousal.

• FALLING ASLEEP •

Falling asleep can be a frightening experience for your baby. We've all felt the strange sensation of becoming aware that you are losing consciousness. Sometimes it's a pleasant, floating feeling, as your book drops from your hand, or noises drift away into a background murmur. But sometimes we startle into full alertness at just this moment, as if there is a primitive reflex at work that tells us it is dangerous to fall asleep until we are sure everything is safe.

For a helpless, totally dependent baby, separation from his parents would once have meant certain death from exposure, hunger or attack by predators. Falling asleep is a particularly risky form of separation. Asleep, we are more vulnerable. It may be some instinctive knowledge of this that makes some babies resist being put down to sleep.

To your baby, the experience of falling asleep may feel as if he is literally falling through the air. Some babies always cry a little as they go through it. Others may be restless, tossing their heads as if they are trying to keep themselves awake. If you consider what falling asleep feels like to you, it will be easier to recognize your baby's needs at this time. He doesn't need to be picked up and woken fully, so that the whole process of getting to sleep has to start all over again. He needs a chance to make the transition from waking to sleep on his own. Once he has been allowed to do that often enough, in an atmosphere of security and reassurance, he learns to trust himself to do it whenever he needs to. The process of falling asleep on his own becomes familiar to him. Most important of all, it becomes his own experience, under his own control. Falling asleep is something we can only do for ourselves, although other people can help. It's the same for your baby.

Our instinct is to do everything for a new baby. We respond to his total dependency by feeling he can do nothing for himself. But given the breast, or a bottle, he can suck his food. And given the right conditions, he can fall asleep. Even before your baby is born, think of his sleep as something that he needs and wants for himself, and that you can help him do it until he has learned to manage it on his own.

• BORN TO SLEEP •

While you are expecting your baby, you can lay the foundations for sound sleep habits that will last his whole life. He will be born into a sleep programme, as it were. From the very beginning, you can make his experience of sleep consistent and reassuring. And you can pass on your confidence that it is something he will soon be able to do for himself.

He is not going to be in control of his own sleep for some time to come. The ability to keep himself awake at will doesn't develop until late in the first year, around nine months. He is born with absolutely no idea of what is expected of him; no ideas at all, really, beyond the survival instinct that makes him lunge for the nipple and resist separation from his parents.

At first you are in control of your baby's sleep. That doesn't mean you can make him sleep. It means you are the one with the knowledge and understanding of what sleep means to your baby, so you are the one who can give him what he needs to sleep well. Gradually you will be handing control of his sleep over to your baby, as he begins to learn the skills and confidence to manage it for himself.

SLEEP PLAN FOR PREGNANCY

▶ Sit down, calm down, stop and think. What will your new baby really need? What will you really need? Sleep helps your baby adjust to life outside the womb and helps you adjust to becoming a parent.

▶ Think about your own sleep habits. Consider that you will unconsciously pass on your own attitudes to your baby.

▶ When preparing for sleep yourself, think about what sleep will mean to your baby, and how you plan to help him sleep well from the start.

▶ Notice your own sleep needs – to be relaxed, to feel safe and secure, how it is difficult to go back to sleep if something is worrying you. Imagine your baby with the same needs.

▶ Don't dwell on the broken nights to come. Think of them as a brief stage in the process of how your baby learns to sleep.

▶ Think of yourself as being in control of your baby's sleep until he can manage it for himself. Gradually you will be handing control of his sleep over to your baby.

2

WHOSE SLEEP IS IT ANYWAY?
Focus on Parents

'I feel I'm only now really getting to know her, getting closely involved with her in the way that her mother has been from the start. Perhaps it's because she spent the nine months of pregnancy connected to our baby, and I needed that much time to catch up.'

Father of Naomi, aged nine months.

HELPING your new baby to sleep well is one of the first things you will have to do as parents. After the decision to breast feed or bottle feed, it is the next big choice. Yet you might think you don't have much choice when it comes to sleep. You know you would like your new baby to sleep well, but perhaps you feel it's a matter of luck. It isn't, as this book shows. There is a tremendous amount you can do to make sure your baby develops good sleep habits from the start. But the thing that can make the biggest difference of all has nothing to do with the baby. It is the way you look after yourself.

• YOU ARE THE WORLD •

Your new baby takes her whole idea of the world from you, and everything you do has an impact on her. As far as she is concerned, the world *is* you. She has little awareness of herself as a separate individual and only a fragmented perception of her environment. You are essential as the provider of food and comfort, but you are much more than that. You are her security, her anchor, her guide in a new and mysterious universe.

This chapter looks at the kind of things that can affect you and make it difficult for you to help your baby sleep. The next one shows how, while trying to help, parents can end up making it impossible for their baby to sleep. Knowing how this can happen is the best way of making sure it doesn't. These two chapters are crucial to the approach of understanding your baby's sleep because, if you are unwittingly preventing her from sleeping, whatever method you use to try to help her sleep stands no chance of success.

• YOU HOLD THE KEY •

The idea that you can make the difference to whether your baby sleeps well or badly is a double-edged sword. It means you can do something about it. You don't have just to hope for the best and muddle through, trusting that things will settle down of their own accord, and wondering what on earth to do when they don't. On the other hand, it is not easy to accept that your baby's sleep problem is really your problem. It might even seem as if your baby's sleep problem is your fault. It isn't. But the fact that your baby is very closely tuned in to you means it is pointless to consider her behaviour in isolation. All sorts of things can affect you without your being aware of it. Indirectly they will also affect your baby. But none of it is your fault. Neither is it the baby's. It's not your partner's fault, or your mother's. It is just what happens.

• YOUR BABY WILL EXPRESS YOUR • FEELINGS

A baby's sleep problem may be the final link in a chain of difficulties in her family. Often it's the place tensions and conflicts show up. Adults can bottle up their feelings, but a baby can't. She will express anything she feels, and one way she does it is by being unable to relax and sleep.

Parents are offered no information on this aspect of their baby's sleep, at least not until they report a sleep problem, which may, by then, be quite severe. This is unfair. You may be doing everything right and giving your baby ideal conditions for establishing sound sleep habits. You may have asked everywhere for advice and nothing has helped.

You can start to feel angry with your baby, or a failure as a parent. At your wits' end, you may simply decide to give up all hope of a decent night's sleep. But the truth is that nothing can solve your child's sleep problem when there is an underlying confusion in your communication with your baby that means she is receiving the wrong signals about sleep.

Parents may be strongly affected by their experiences, but they may not pay themselves enough attention to realize it. What you are feeling sometimes expresses itself through your baby, who will pick up even those emotions and tensions you are unaware of. Her crying, or inability to sleep, may seem to have no obvious cause. But it can have its origins in your own feelings – often feelings stirred up by her arrival in your life.

• BIRTH •

Once a baby is safely born, we are expected to put the birth behind us. A 'good' birth, where everything has gone smoothly and the baby is born healthy, may be taken for granted by families lucky enough to have one. But in fact it makes a big difference to the start of your life with your baby. Your confidence as new parents gets a tremendous boost if the actual experience of becoming parents has been a good one. You bask in a glow of success before you have even started, and your ease and pleasure is communicated to your baby.

A complicated, painful, difficult or frightening birth makes the process of adjustment harder for everyone. It is natural to want to forget a distressing experience when it's over, especially when you have been rewarded with a new baby to focus on instead. But she may be in shock after the trauma of her arrival and so may you. It is very difficult to get to know each other as a new family when everyone involved is traumatized in their own separate way.

An emergency Caeserian section, for example, can leave a mother with conflicting feelings. She is grateful that her baby is safe and well, but on another level she may feel somehow less of a mother for not giving birth naturally. Sometimes these feelings are strongly denied and come out only years later. Both parents may feel shaken and uncertain after coping with unexpected surgery as well as the birth of their baby. If your baby has difficulties immediately after birth, it may seem to you that she needs doctors and nurses more than she needs you. All this will colour the start of your life together, perhaps by making it hard for you to feel close to your baby.

Parents can feel terrible if they don't fall in love with their new baby instantly. There are good reasons why you may not, and it doesn't mean anything in itself – you and your baby may just need a little more time. Feeling bad about it can be more of a problem. You may feel there is something wrong with you, because your reaction was not what you anticipated. Your baby may seem a disappointment, because she did not produce the 'right' response in you.

Even a baby who looks different from the one you imagined while you were pregnant – a different sex, for example – may be a shock to you, and that too means it will take longer to begin the process of getting to know her and accept her as she is.

All these sorts of feelings are likely to be bottled up and barely acknowledged in the eventful first few days and weeks. But if they are there, even if they're ignored, they are part of your relationship with your baby, and that can make it harder to get in tune with her and her needs. The whole business of looking after your baby can seem to get off on the wrong foot.

• BECOMING A PARENT •

Quite apart from the birth itself, becoming a parent is a shock. The so-called 'baby blues', the weepy feeling a few days after childbirth, is invariably put down to hormones. But it should also be recognized as a perfectly natural and appropriate reaction to the momentous experience you've been through. People do feel shaky or tearful once the initial shock of a crisis has worn off, and having a baby is no exception.

Becoming a parent is a massive shift in your own identity. From the time you were born, your life has been geared towards independence and responsibility for yourself. Suddenly that whole process is turned on its head. With the birth of your baby, you become completely responsible for someone else, someone who depends on you for her very survival. As a person you have created and brought into the world, she is the first to have an unconditional claim on you.

Whatever age you are when this happens, it marks the defining moment when you become an adult. Overnight, you're not the younger generation any more. Yesterday you were your parents' child. Today you are someone's parent as well. The child-like part of you has to take more of a back seat; the adult part has to play a much bigger role than before.

Some parents achieve this transition easily and naturally. Others find it a real struggle. Some recognize it and laugh, like the father of a four-month-old boy who grew his hair long, bought a Hell's Angels leather jacket and threatened to join a motorcycle club. 'I'm competing with the baby for attention,' he acknowledged ruefully. 'I don't want to be middle aged and boring just because I'm a dad. I want to be wild, and young and free.'

Parenthood brings out a new dimension, for better or worse, in everyone it happens to. The thing that seems to make the biggest difference is how ready you are to embrace change. Expectant parents who insist the new baby will make no difference to their lives are in for a tough time, because they are resisting what is going to happen to them anyway. Those who anticipate a big shift on all fronts, and actually look forward to it, seem to enjoy the transformation of their lives.

Having a baby is an identity crisis. You know you're a parent now – but that's just a label. What does it mean to the unique individual that is you? Only by living through it can you find out. This impact on your deepest sense of yourself is a serious shock to your system.

• LACK OF SLEEP •

It is very difficult for anyone in a house containing a new-born baby to get an unbroken night's sleep. On top of that there's little chance to catch up on rest and adjust to the momentous event of becoming a parent. A new father may have to go back to work within days. A new mother may not have any help at home.

Lack of the lighter, dreaming or REM stage of sleep, in particular, affects our concentration, as well as our ability to remain optimistic and cheerful. Unfortunately these are exactly the qualities you need to listen and respond to your baby, and to reassure her that all is well in this strange new world.

It helps to be aware that lack of sleep can, in itself, cause feelings of confusion and hopelessness. It also helps to catch up with whatever rest you can. It is easy to get things out of perspective and start frantic activity every time you put the baby down. Remember that work can be a way of avoiding your feelings. Don't waste this important time on inessentials. Eat convenience food. Give up housework. Put things off, let things slide. For a week or two, it doesn't matter. You, your relationship with your partner and your baby do.

If any help is available, try to direct it towards the ironing, cleaning and cooking. Some grandmothers can be persuaded to take over the kitchen. Offers to take the baby off your hands are well meant and you will be grateful for the odd break. But these early days are an investment in your relationship with your baby. They are the time to start getting to know each other as a family. The more time you spend with your new baby, the sooner you will know the meaning of her different noises; and therefore the sooner she will trust you to meet her needs and start to feel secure in her world.

• YOUR OWN BABYHOOD •

New parents are at an emotionally vulnerable stage. Your baby's total dependence, and the urgency of her demands, churn up feelings you may not recognize, to do with the way you were cared for when you were dependent and needy yourself.

Having a baby takes you back to the time when you were a baby. You will find you have certain responses to your baby that feel instinctive or automatic. These have their roots in your own experience of childhood. You might find yourself singing lullabies that you didn't know you knew, or talking to your baby in a particular way, only to find that your mother talks to the baby in exactly the same way.

The way you care for your baby echoes the way you were looked after yourself. One of the most difficult problems a new parent can have to cope with is when these automatic responses conflict with the kind of parent you want to be. Say, for example, you feel you should have been picked up and cuddled more as a baby. You may be determined that you will be different: your baby will gets lots of cuddles. You actively want to do the opposite of what you feel happened to you. Yet, when your baby cries, you find yourself worrying that if you pick her up, you might spoil her. This is an automatic response. It feels natural to you, while the way that you have decided to handle your baby may not.

The same process can work in another way. Again, say your childhood left you with a feeling that you didn't get enough attention. Because of this, you jump to console and cuddle your baby every time she cries. But you may be thinking of the baby you once were, rather than of the one you have now. She probably feels that she gets plenty of attention. What she may need from you is a sign of your confidence in her to manage on her own.

• YOUR RELATIONSHIP WITH YOUR • PARTNER

Everything seems to revolve around a new baby, and the needs of new parents are easily overlooked. Fathers, especially, often get no attention at all – no wonder they bottle up their feelings. Some new mothers and fathers understand each other very well, and support each other as they adjust to life as a new family. Sometimes, though, the experience of becoming parents affects two people quite differently, and they react in ways that open up a gulf of misunderstanding between them. It is vital to keep the channels of communication with your partner open when there is so much going on.

'WHEN our baby, Naomi, was a few weeks old,' says Michelle, 'Dan told me he felt as if I had gone away from him. I didn't have the energy to talk in the evenings. When the baby was asleep, I just wanted to rest, read, and be by myself for a while, after meeting her needs all day. But I knew it was part of the process of adjusting, and my way of looking after myself as well as the baby.

'I told him everything would be fine, and there was nothing to worry about. I said all he had to do was be there for us. He was concerned, but I was not, so I felt I should take the lead to reassure him. But I was also aware I was relying on him to have the confidence to trust me, and follow my lead. I believed he would, and he did.'

Parents can be a great support to each other in their own experiences as well as in helping their new baby feel secure, so she can quickly settle into regular rhythms of eating and sleeping. But it sometimes happens that parents come from families where babies are managed in quite different ways. Although this may never have cropped up in their relationship before, when they have a baby of their own, they find they have very different ideas about what is best. The result can be arguments and tension at exactly the time when everyone needs most understanding, support and reassurance. Again, the best course of action is to try to bring these experiences of your own out into the open and acknowledge them. Strong family habits and assumptions build up around even little things, like what a baby's first food should be or how she is dressed. Whether your baby wears her mittens or not really doesn't matter. What does matter is a feeling of harmony around her.

• YOUR PARENTS •

Your relationship with your own parents also changes when you have a baby. There is a big shift in everyone's roles, as you become parents and they become grandparents. Sometimes this is a difficult transition. Your parents may find it hard to take a back seat and hand over the parenting job to you. They may not feel ready to be grandparents, with the new identity that means for them. Or they may not be able to answer your questions and help you in the way you would like.

Having your own baby stirs up new feelings about your parents. You may respect them more, realizing for the first time what they went through, and what a good job they did looking after you. Or you may feel, perhaps for the first time, that they were inadequate parents in some way. Sometimes this causes underlying tension and resentment, even when things are all right on the surface.

You might feel upset or resentful if you need your parents and they are not around, for one reason or another. There is evidence that mothers whose own mothers die before their babies are born are more likely to have babies with sleep problems. Perhaps the absence of their own mother's support in their new role as a mother makes them less confident and less able to reassure their baby.

• ANGER •

You may be angry with your baby for all sorts of reasons. Perhaps the birth was a difficult one and you see your baby as the cause of your shock and distress; or you might resent her for getting so much love and attention, if you feel you aren't getting enough yourself. It can even be infuriating to try to soothe her when she cries, when you feel like crying yourself! Especially when you are short of sleep, and more likely to get things out of perspective, you may become furious with your partner, or your own parents. Trying to avoid a scene with them may mean your angry feelings are expressed in your dealings with your baby. It's not unusual to have moments when you even feel you hate your baby.

These feelings are only natural. Don't feel guilty when you have them, and don't bottle them up because you think they are 'wrong'. The best thing to do is express them to someone not too emotionally involved, perhaps an understanding friend or your health visitor. You may well find yourself crying: 'I'm so tired, and she woke up five times last night, and she's cried half the day, and I just hate her!' Every parent has these feelings at times. It's important to remember that they are only feelings, and quite understandable. Often just being able to describe how you feel is such a relief that you are able to laugh about it a few minutes later.

Having a shoulder to cry on is a safety valve. It lets you acknowledge your own stresses and strains, and frees you to start feeling loving again. If you ever feel that your anger is in danger of getting out of control, it is absolutely essential to tell a responsible person for your baby's sake.

• KEEP YOURSELF IN FOCUS •

The answer to all these potential pitfalls is to try to be aware of them. Once you find ways of thinking about your own feelings, your own needs and experiences, it becomes possible to separate them from your dealings with your baby. This can have the effect of setting your baby free to sleep. It can be a relief for her to be no longer entangled in your anxieties.

To do this it is vital to keep yourself in sharp focus. Your baby is part of you, and she thinks you are part of her. But you are not. Your baby is important, but not more important than you. In one way she is less important. Her needs are simpler: if she feels warm, well fed, loved and secure, she is fine. She doesn't have a long and complex history that needs to be taken into account.

And the job you have to do is even bigger than the one she has, adjusting to the world. You make it possible for her to do it. She can't do it without you. You are having to be everything to her, at the same time as adjusting yourself, your relationship with your partner and your family to your new status as parents, and recovering from the experience of childbirth. It's a tall order.

Your baby knows how to make her presence felt and her needs clear. Although it's easy to feel pushed into the background, it is better to keep your own needs in mind too, because you need to take care of yourself as well as the baby, for your baby's sake as much as your own. It needn't be a conflict over who comes first. It is more a question of being aware of your needs, considering your baby's and trying to balance them so that nobody is deprived. Looking after yourself makes it less likely that your baby will absorb conflicts and tensions that could interfere with her sleep.

You and your baby are closely connected, so that your feelings and behaviour affect her as much as hers affect you. It should feel like a two-way relationship, not an unrelenting drain on you with nothing being put back. The only way you can achieve that is by not losing sight of yourself.

You can't help your feelings. But recognizing that they *are* your feelings, and why you have them, is liberating. It frees you from a fruitless cycle of blaming everyone else, and seeking solutions everywhere, and lets you begin to find some answers of your own. It lets you deal with your feelings and leaves your baby free to get on with sleeping and growing.

SLEEP PLAN FOR FOCUS ON PARENTS

▶ Look after yourself, for your baby's sake as well as your own.

▶ Try to work out any sources of conflict and tension in yourself that might be communicated to your baby. If you are angry, talk to someone about it. Your feelings are important.

▶ When thinking about your baby, think about yourself as well. Remember that you are her whole world.

▶ Try to compensate for broken nights with extra rest and relaxation, and make allowances for yourself when you are short of sleep.

► If help is available, try to use it to spend more relaxed time with your baby. It's an investment in your relationship.

► Recognize the impact of the birth, and of the experience of becoming parents.

► Acknowledge your own feelings, and accept and understand your partner's, even if they are different from yours.

► Don't blame anyone, especially not yourself.

3
LET ME SLEEP
How to Stop Your Baby Sleeping

'We originally planned to have him sleep in our bed.
But he slept so badly it was impossible. He was no
better in his cot in our room. We tried everything –
sleep programmes, the works. Finally I said: 'That's
it, he's got to sleep in another room.' That was a
month ago. And he's slept all night ever since.'

Mother of Zachary, aged one.

WHILE DOING your best to give your baby the best
possible care, you can care too much. You can do too
much for him, pay him too much attention, respond to him too
fully. It can get to the point where you are doing everything for
him except leave him alone. And that may be what he needs.

The title of this chapter is slightly tongue in cheek, of course:
nobody really intends to stop their baby sleeping. But it is easily
done without your meaning to do it, and the effect is the same as
if you deliberately set out to interfere with your baby's sleep.
Sometimes the hardest thing to do is nothing at all. And sometimes nothing is exactly what needs to be done.

When a baby cries, we assume he needs our help. And
sometimes he does. But sometimes he doesn't. There is a cry that
says: 'Help me sleep.' It comes from a baby who is uncomfortable, or who needs reassurance.

But there is also a cry that says: 'Let me sleep.' It comes from a baby who feels his parents' presence so strongly that he can't relax into the solitude of sleep. Instead of being reassured by his parents' attention, this baby is over-stimulated by it.

How does it happen that parents stop their babies sleeping? No parent *wants* their baby to wake several times a night, or for bedtime to become a drawn-out, exhausting struggle. Nobody wants a baby to sleep more than parents who may not have had an unbroken night for a year. Yet a tangle of tensions can grow up between you and your baby that makes sleep impossible.

Your feelings, attitudes, beliefs and habits shape the way you relate to your baby, as was explained in Chapter 2. Although your baby is born biologically adapted to gradually becoming able to sleep all night, the process can easily be thrown off course or delayed. If he gets clear signals that night-time is when we sleep, that his world is a safe, secure place and that his parents trust him to manage without them until morning, he will sleep much better than a baby who doesn't get those signals.

• Night Feeding •

One of the commonest reasons for a baby to wake at night is when night feeding is continued beyond when he physically needs it. This will make it impossible for him to consolidate his sleep into one long, unbroken stretch.

The relationship between food and sleep is discussed in detail in Chapter 6. Here, while we are considering the way your influence on your baby can prevent him sleeping, we will look at just one example. It is important to understand how this can happen because, just as no one actively wants to keep their child awake, no one feeds their baby without believing he needs feeding. He may, or he may not. The point is that when you believe he does, it can blind you to his signals that food is not the solution. Indeed it may be the problem.

——— ★★★ ———

PAULA felt strongly that her own mother had not been the kind of mother she would have liked her to be. She felt that she had been too caught up in her own concerns, and not particularly understanding of Paula as a child. Paula was determined that she would be a different kind of mother. She wanted to be there for her children and in touch with their needs.

Paula responded to any cry from her babies in the night by feeding them. Throughout both her babies' first year, they cried for their feed several times a night. Their disturbed sleep made them irritable in the daytime, and their appetites were poor after so much milk at night. That was no surprise. The mystery was why Paula continued to feed her babies at night, when she knew they were old enough not to need it.

We can guess that it satisfied Paula's need to be an attentive, involved mother, in a way she felt she had missed out on as a baby herself. Her way of comforting her babies when they cried was with food, a symbol of good mothering in our society. Although her babies' need was for sleep, Paula couldn't see this clearly while she was preoccupied with her own impulses. Her instinct was to feed them. She needed to feel different from her mother, and getting up for her babies in the night was one way of meeting that need of hers.

The important thing is that Paula *thought* she was doing the best thing for her babies. The dramatic improvement in her babies' well-being after the feedings stopped and they could sleep all night proved that sleep was what they had needed all along. But when you are caught up in instinctive habits and attitudes of your own, it can be difficult to see your baby as a person with his own, distinct needs, quite separate from yours.

★★★

• YOUR NEEDS AND YOUR BABY'S •

Paula's experience shows how tightly woven the threads of a baby's sleep problem can be. She was preventing her babies from sleeping, but she believed that she was meeting their needs. Feeding them felt like the right thing to do. And that, in turn, had its roots in her feelings about her own childhood. Luckily, unravelling the tangle is usually much simpler than the way you got into it. All Paula had to do was stop feeding her babies at night. They could then sleep without waking for the feeds they had come to expect. And Paula was freed to consider her own feelings in peace, while her babies slept.

This kind of muddle can grow up around all sorts of things. It starts in a parent's feelings, and ends in a sleep problem.

Parents who are out at work all day naturally want to make the most of time with their baby in the evening, and sometimes when he wakes in the middle of the night too. If your baby goes to bed late, or if you play with him when he wakes at night, you may be meeting your own need to be with your baby. You may feel that your baby needs the time with you too. In such a case your baby won't be able to establish a really sound sleep pattern, since some of his daytime behaviour will be carried over into time when he could be sleeping a long, unbroken night. But if you do make this choice, it's best to see it as a definite choice, and be positive and honest about it. It's better for him to go to bed later, having had some happy time with you, than for the two of you to get locked into a struggle over a bedtime you have mixed feelings about. That way there will be no conflict over sleep, and it will be easier to help your baby catch up on sleep when he can. He may benefit from a long morning nap, for example.

Sometimes all that needs to be done is to acknowledge your own feelings and deal with them separately from your baby. This allows you to concentrate on what he is telling you he really needs, instead of on what you think he needs.

• HOW YOUR BABY PICKS UP • TENSION FROM YOU

To sleep well, your baby needs to be comfortable, well fed and relaxed. To relax, he needs to feel safe and secure. This bit is often left out, which makes parents feel, once their baby is fed and comfortable, that he ought to be able to sleep. Then they're understandably mystified and frustrated when he doesn't.

It may be because he feels unsafe. Because you are his world, if he senses tension or conflict in you, his world is out of step. It is not that your thoughts are communicated, as if by telepathy, to your baby. It's simpler than that. Even if you're not thinking about how you feel, anxiety produces tension in your body. Your baby feels the tension as you hold him, and it makes him uneasy.

He can't relax and enjoy his feed. He may pull away from you and feed in an awkward position. He will end up with an unsatisfying feed and perhaps cry from a combination of indigestion, hunger and anxiety. He won't be able to settle to sleep. A small baby's emotions are inseparable from his physical processes, and he will express them through disturbances in his sleep or feeding.

It's also worth remembering that the chemical makeup of his mother's emotions is familiar to him from the womb. The rush of adrenalin in your system when you have a fright makes your unborn baby's beat faster. Endorphins, the chemicals that give us a sensation of well-being, are also shared with your unborn baby. Your baby literally takes part in your emotional states before he's born.

As a new-born baby, he will continue to recognize your skin and your smell. He will immediately sense panic, for example, with its strong adrenalin component. If you feel fearful or uneasy about handling him, he may pick up chemical warning signals that he is in danger. Coming on top of the tension he feels in your body, the stress may be more than he can bear.

Bathtime is a good example. If you feel anxious holding your slippery new baby in the water, he feels altogether unsafe, even though there is nothing more seriously wrong in his world than a nervous parent. To him that is a world without security, and reason enough to panic. He is likely to scream, which will do nothing for your confidence. A good way around this is to take your baby into the bath with you, where holding him against your body makes both of you feel more secure.

In general, relaxing yourself will make an enormous difference to how your baby feels and behaves. Before you pick him up, shake the tension from your arms and hands, and roll your shoulders and neck. Take a few deep breaths. Before you settle down to feed your baby, take an extra minute to make sure that you are comfortable, with your back well supported. Drop your shoulders. Bring your baby towards your body – don't lean forward to him. Check during the feed that your shoulders are still dropped down and free of tension.

• TRUSTING YOUR BABY TO SLEEP •

Your baby needs your help to feel secure. To relax into sleep, he needs to feel it's safe to drop his guard. If he doesn't get this message from you, he will feel too wary and anxious to let go and sleep.

You yourself might not really believe that it is safe to leave your baby to sleep. If you don't believe he can manage without you until morning, he won't be able to. The whole atmosphere of tension around sleep will worry him, and make him even more wakeful and uneasy. Practical ways of dealing with anxiety over your sleeping baby are discussed in the next chapter, on the first weeks of life. Here we are considering how your own experience can indirectly lead to your baby being unable to sleep.

Feeling that it is not safe to let your baby sleep has its roots in your own life. If you have experienced loss or painful separation yourself, putting your baby down and separating from him for the night may stir up those painful feelings. That can send confusing messages to your baby: while you're *telling* him it's time to go to sleep, he's *feeling* the emotional truth of your conflict and uncertainty. Your manner, your tone of voice and the tension in your body all carry stronger signals than anything you actually say or do. He looks to you to tell him what is safe and what is not. If you're not sure about something, he can't feel any trust in it himself.

If you are really anxious, your baby is likely to wake to check that you are all right. Remember that you are his world. If he feels his world is under some kind of threat, he understandably needs to make sure it's still there when he stirs in the night.

Sometimes this is caused by a crisis in the family. When you are very upset, it is difficult to stay in tune with your baby. Your preoccupation with your own feelings means you have no time to think about him or listen carefully to him. Your baby's sleep will probably settle down again when the crisis has passed.

• CONFIDENCE •

Just as frequently, though, there is no catastrophe behind the buildup of anxiety. It may simply be that something is undermining your confidence. Taking care of a baby is an enormous responsibility. Getting to know your baby is a complex process too, especially if this is your first and you are learning all the basics of caring for a baby at the same time. No wonder your confidence is sometimes a bit shaky.

It's important to remember that you need support and reassurance as much as your baby does, and for his sake as much as your own. It is part of what you need to look after your baby. Don't hesitate to ask for it.

Confidence also builds quickly when you can clear your mind of other thoughts and concentrate on listening to your baby's cries, so as to try to work out what they mean. It takes your mind off your own anxiety, and it helps your baby feel understood and reassured.

• WHEN YOUR BABY CRIES •

When your baby cries, try to avoid worrying about what might be wrong. Deliberately adopt a calm, cheerful tone of voice. Acknowledge that he is upset, but don't make it a big deal. A crying baby will close his eyes and shut himself off. It is much easier to work out what is bothering him if you can get him to open his eyes and reconnect with you. Often, directly appealing to him won't work, but taking his attention away from the two of you will. So you might say something like this:

'I understand you're upset. Don't worry. We'll sort it out. Oh look! I can see a cat. Look at the cat!'

Make cat noises, lift him up high – whatever it takes to distract him into opening his eyes. That breaks the cycle of the two of you feeding on each other's tension, and brings him back from the incoherent state he's got himself into. Once he's a bit calmer, you'll be able to tell whether he's hot, or tired, or cross, or whatever.

If he keeps working himself up and you start to feel tense, it helps to put him down somewhere safe, go out of the room, take a few deep breaths and remind yourself that there is nothing really wrong, with you or your baby. You can then go back in a calmer frame of mind to convey this message to him. Taking him outside will sometimes make him stop crying instantly. If distraction doesn't work, you could just sit very calmly with him in a quiet, dim room. Whatever you do, try to avoid being infected by his anxiety. It's not easy. But the cooler you are, the sooner he'll realize there's no cause for alarm.

As one mother of four put it: 'With the last one, I'm so laid back, I find myself saying to him: "I know you're upset, but I've got to go to bed." '

• CONSISTENCY •

Your baby is learning the way the world works from you. If you feel uncertain about what is best for him, the way you care for him is likely to be inconsistent. One day you might pick him up whenever he cries; the next you worry that you are spoiling him, and leave him to cry. This confuses your baby. It makes it impossible for him to build up a picture of the world as a dependable place, in which he can begin to relax. He will find it hard to sleep, because he will be constantly wondering what's going to happen next, and experimenting to see if he can find out.

That's why a regular bedtime routine works so well. It sends clear, definite signals about how the world works: sleep follows bed, which follows bath. It makes him feel secure, and he needs to feel secure to go to sleep content and stay asleep all night.

While your baby is too young for a bedtime routine, you can achieve the same effect by being very consistent. Babies respond well to a degree of repetition that most adults find tedious. On a night when he decides to test your consistency, it's worth remembering that however many times you tuck him up and say good night, it's not as tedious as a baby who gets the idea that night-time is playtime.

• SEPARATION AND INDEPENDENCE •

Sleeping well is a sign of your baby's growing independence. Many parents feel a kind of shock when their baby first sleeps through the night. It can be hard to believe that this tiny infant, who has dominated your nights for weeks on end, can suddenly manage alone.

Sometimes, even while you long for your baby to sleep, letting him achieve this independence is difficult. He will never again need you as simply, obviously and constantly as he did when he cried for food every few hours.

Even while enjoying your baby's progress, it's natural to have feelings of sadness as he leaves baby stages behind him. Some part of you may want to keep him a baby as long as possible, especially if you expect him to be your last, or only, baby. There is something impressively grown-up and self-sufficient about a baby who grins good night and burbles good morning. It can be unnerving. If you find it hard to accept that your baby doesn't need you for as long as twelve hours every night, he will sense that you want him to wake up.

──────── ★★★ ────────

At fifteen months, Alice, the baby of the family and the only girl, was still waking several times a night, and taking up to an hour to settle each time. She was not yet walking, and every meal turned into a battle to persuade her to swallow a spoonful or two. On holiday her father noticed Alice's friend of the same age cheerfully munching her way through family meals, brandishing a fork.

'Let's not give Alice baby food any more,' he said. 'And let's stop spoon-feeding her. If her friend can eat proper food by herself, so can Alice.'

The transformation was dramatic. Alice was delighted with her new finger foods, and she started walking the very same day. Within a week she slept through the night.

'I think she was just fed up with being treated like a baby,' said her father.

In showing he had confidence in Alice to eat without help, her father also gave her the confidence to take a great leap towards independence by walking, and by sleeping all night. Until then all the messages she had received reinforced the idea that she could not manage on her own.

It is interesting that this happened on holiday, when Alice's father had more time with the family. Alice had got into a vicious circle. The crosser she got, the more she was babied, and the crosser she got. Her father's fresh perspective on all this provided a much-needed breakthrough.

★★★

• UNDOING THE TANGLE •

It is often the most loving, concerned, devoted parents whose babies can't seem to sleep through the night. You can try too hard. It can be more helpful to relax and trust your baby to sleep through the night as soon as he is able to do it.

When he stirs in the night, don't be too quick to assume that he needs you. When your baby is restless and finding it hard to settle, you naturally want to do everything in your power to help him. But your efforts may be exactly what is keeping your baby awake. Especially when you are tired and stressed yourself, an atmosphere of tension is quickly created.

Sometimes parents are driven to desperate measures. You may be so relieved to find something that works that you resort to doing it every night – only to find that your baby refuses, sometimes for years, to go to sleep on his own. One little boy of two and a half was driven around in the family car for an hour or so every night until he fell asleep – and it's not that uncommon. A 'solution' like this is a disaster for parents. It ruins your evening and creates extra stress at exactly the time you most need to relax and have some time to yourselves. It's pretty dreadful for babies too. No baby really wants to be driven around in the car all evening. It's just that it has become the only way he knows how to go to sleep. What he needs is to learn how to go to sleep in peace and quiet on his own. Basically he needs parents who are less willing to devote themselves to him.

Your baby is important, but no more important than anyone

else. Don't fall into the trap of putting him in charge of what happens in the whole household. Life inevitably revolves around a new baby at first. But he will quickly settle down, given encouragement. Babies who have to fit in to an existing family are often calmer and easier, simply because less fuss is made of them.

• PICK HIM UP OR LEAVE HIM • TO CRY?

Another reason for babies being overwhelmed by attention is our rejection of the idea, widespread in the 1950s and 1960s, that picking up a baby when he cries will spoil him. You still hear it: 'You are making a rod for your own back, picking up that baby all the time. He'll never learn.'

To most modern parents, leaving a baby to cry seems cruel. We rightly see no reason why a baby who needs food or comfort should be left alone to howl. But that shouldn't mean rushing to pick him up every time he opens his mouth: it just makes it impossible for him to settle down.

The picture is complicated by the fact that today's parents may have been left to cry as babies themselves, by parents following the advice of their day. As Chapter 2 showed, this can leave a legacy of mixed feelings. We don't want to leave a baby to cry, as perhaps we feel we were left. On the other hand, we may have a deep-seated suspicion that picking him up will, indeed, spoil him.

This conflict sends confusing messages to your baby. Sometimes he will be picked up, sometimes left to cry. Or he may be picked up by a parent who feels anxious and uncertain that it is the right thing to do. Your baby will sense this and find it even harder to calm down.

Meeting your baby's needs includes leaving him in peace when that's what he needs. You can satisfy him without indulging his every whim. In practice this means giving a small baby all the contact and closeness he asks for, while still encouraging him to go to sleep on his own.

There is evidence that babies who are carried and cuddled a

lot in their early months go on to be better sleepers than others. Perhaps these babies have had their early need for comfort and reassurance met in full, and this has helped them to feel safe in their world, and able to relax and sleep.

Meeting your baby's need for reassurance is not the same thing as spoiling him. Being spoilt means getting everything you want, whether you need it or not. A new baby only knows what he needs: love, security, food and sleep. Part of the process of adjusting to your life together is discovering how best to meet these needs for your particular baby. However you do it, you are not spoiling him. You can't, until he is old enough to want things he doesn't need.

You can, however, confuse him. He may not want things he doesn't need, but we often find it difficult to work out what he does need. We sometimes give him food when he isn't hungry, stimulation when he needs peace, or ignore him when he needs human contact. We sometimes pick him up when what he needs is to go to sleep.

We do it because his behaviour can be mystifying, and our own instincts sometimes get in the way. To break a pattern of confusion, step back a bit from your baby. Don't feel you have to do something the minute he cries. You will not be leaving him to cry. That means ignoring him. What you will be doing is exactly the opposite. You will be watching and listening to him, so that you can work out what he is feeling and find the most appropriate response.

SLEEP PLAN FOR LETTING YOUR BABY SLEEP

▶ Consider your own feelings and experiences. Try to deal with them separately from your baby.

▶ Check that your body is loose and relaxed before you pick up or feed your baby.

▶ Remember that you are as important as your baby, and you

need support and reassurance in order to look after him. Don't hesitate to ask for it.

▶ Trust your baby to manage on his own when he is peaceful or asleep. You will be encouraging his independence.

▶ Try not to let your baby pick up anxiety from you. Deliberately put on a calm, cheerful voice when he cries, and reassure him that you will sort it out together.

▶ Remember the baby has his problems, and you have yours. Try not to get distressed when he is.

▶ If you feel tension building up, distract yourself and your baby by going outside or looking at something interesting together. If all else fails, go into another room for a minute and take a few deep breaths to calm down.

▶ Try to be consistent. However repetitive it is for you, it is reassuring for your baby.

▶ Be as positive as you can. Try to reinforce your own confidence, and assure your baby that you have complete confidence in him.

4

EARLY NIGHTS
The First Weeks

'My first baby never seemed to sleep, but it was my fault. I didn't think he could make it through the night. With this one, I leave her in peace, and she sleeps.'

Mother of Isabella, three months, and Carlos, nine.

H UMAN babies are born the most immature of all species. A new-born baby has only a quarter of her adult brain volume. If a baby's head grew any more in the womb, it wouldn't fit through her mother's pelvis. So your baby arrives in the world not quite ready to take part in it. Helpless, vulnerable and totally dependent, she needs your complete care and protection as she makes the transition to fully fledged babyhood.

Your baby's immaturity at birth is central to an understanding of how sleep patterns develop. Major shifts in her brain function are going on in the early months. We recognize this when we say a new-born baby is 'just a scrap of humanity', but by three months she has become 'a proper baby'. These different stages of development each have their own, quite distinct needs. In effect you are dealing with a different baby.

When your baby is just a few days or weeks old, you can't expect any predictable pattern of sleep. This is not the time for a bedtime routine, or changing into pyjamas. But that doesn't mean there is nothing you can do at this stage. Far from it. You can help your baby learn good sleep habits from the day she is born, and she will show the first signs of sleeping all night as early as one month old. This chapter covers three key areas where you can make an enormous contribution, in the first days and weeks of life, to your baby's adaptation to sleeping all night. They are:

- the hunger cry;
- learning to go to sleep;
- the core night.

Just as it would be wrong to think there is nothing you can do at this stage, remember you can also do too much. Continuing to offer night feeds to a baby who no longer needs them, for example, will make it impossible for her to consolidate her sleep into an unbroken night. Rocking her, or feeding her, until she is sound asleep will prevent her from learning to go to sleep on her own.

Your baby is biologically programmed to adapt to sleeping all night. Your aim is to encourage that process. To a large extent that means not interfering with it. It can also mean letting her find her own way, even if it's not the way you expected.

• MEETING YOUR BABY'S NEEDS •

Babies do seem to have very definite ideas about what they need. Some are peaceful from the start. They are able to use sleep to escape the constant stimulation of their environment. Others are hyper-sensitive and anxious at first, and need lots of help to settle down. If yours is one of these, you may be reassured by findings that babies who are held and carried a lot in their early days go on to be better sleepers than others.

Whatever your particular baby's needs, you can be confident that you can meet them while still sending her the clear message that night-time is for sleeping.

On the other hand, resisting a new baby's demands for your attention can sometimes have the effect of making her more demanding over a long period. It is as if early frustration creates persistent neediness and dissatisfaction.

———— ★★★ ————

Tom, aged three and a half weeks, was fretting miserably in his lean-back chair.

'He needs to sleep,' said his aunt, a mother of three.

'No,' said his mother, 'he doesn't sleep in the daytime any more.'

His aunt ignored this and lay Tom across her knee, patting his back. He quickly quietened and went to sleep.

'Well' said his mother, 'of course he'll sleep if you sit with him on your knee all day. I haven't got time for that.'

Now aged almost two, Tom still wakes several times a night, demanding to see his mother before he'll go back to sleep.

———— ★★★ ————

A new baby's needs can seem extreme, but who are we to decide what a new baby may need? We can't remember what adjustment to life outside the womb feels like. Your baby has a tremendous task on her hands. Even when she is just a few days old, there is something you can do that will make an enormous difference to how quickly she settles into good sleep patterns.

• THE HUNGER CRY •

The hunger cry is the first thing to learn about your new baby. Because sleep is inseparable from food at first, the cry that carries your baby's hunger signal is very important – so that you can tell when she's not hungry, as much as when she is. That's how you know when she needs something other than food. This, in turn, is the first step towards finding other ways to settle her at night, and avoid encouraging a habit of night feeding that will prevent her sleeping through the night.

It may seem simpler to offer the breast or bottle, letting your baby refuse it if she's not hungry. But babies enjoy sucking for its own sake, and very often take food when it's offered, even when they're not hungry. This can cause indigestion, as well as confusion over both food and sleep. They can't establish regular body rhythms, and it's difficult for them to begin the process of learning how to recognize what they want.

This is a trap I fell into, and from which Lucy had to dig me out. My baby got peckish, and I promptly fed her. The result was that she was never hungry enough to take a really good feed, and her tummy was never full enough for her to settle down for a long sleep. She would doze off at the breast and then protest when put down to sleep.

'Give her a bottle,' advised one doctor. 'The milk is delivered faster, so her tummy will fill up without her having to work so hard for it.' But I didn't want to give up breast feeding, and Lucy convinced me I didn't have to. She showed me how to make sure that my baby was really hungry before I fed her and to try other methods of soothing her if she wasn't.

'Listen for a particular note in her cry,' Lucy said. 'It's a sharper, more urgent sound. Not whimpering or complaining or protesting, but a cry that seems to say: "Feed me NOW!"'.

Once you think you have a hungry baby, you can confirm it by testing the 'rooting reflex'. If you stroke the baby's cheek, she will lunge towards that side as if her life depended on it.

If your baby seems unhappy rather than hungry, it is tempting to offer food for comfort. The drawback to this is that your baby will start to use you as a comfort object. Allowing it at night can start a lasting habit of waking for feeding. 'Remember,' Lucy would say, 'Mummy is not a dummy.'

From the day you bring her home from the hospital, you are helping your baby towards being able to sleep all night when you concentrate on the signals she sends and try to sort out their meaning. It's not always easy. Indigestion may feel just like hunger pains to your baby, so her cry may sound the same. But when you stop to listen to her you are breaking the automatic assumption that a crying baby needs to be fed.

• SETTLING A RESTLESS BABY: WHAT • TO DO INSTEAD OF FEEDING

Once you have ruled out hunger, one or more of these tried-and-tested methods will help soothe an uncomfortable baby:

- Go outside. This can have an almost magical effect. It may be the sudden change of air, but crying will often stop as if it had been switched off.

- Walk with her. Experiment with how the baby likes to be held as you walk. Some babies like to hang right over your shoulder. The pressure on their tummies may help with indigestion.

- Swaddle your baby firmly in a shawl or flannel cot sheet. Lie her on it, wrap first one side then the other quite tightly over her chest, including her arms, then tuck up the feet, so that the baby is a neat parcel. Perhaps this reminds her of the way she was contained by the womb. But it must be firm – loose wrappings can irritate her.

- Lie her face down over your knee and pat her back.

- Prop her up on your knees and talk to her, with your face about 12 inches from hers – the perfect distance for her to practise focusing.

- Show her interesting things. The washing machine is popular. So are waving leaves, dancing mobiles and playing children.

- Sing to her, or play music.

- Dance with her if she's bored. If she's irritable, however, it may make it worse.

- Remove a warm layer. Babies get very uncomfortable when they are hot, especially in snowsuits in overheated shops. They haven't yet developed the ability to regulate their own temperature, as we do.

- Sit in a rocking chair with her: it may be soothing for you both.

- Consider using a dummy. Some new babies are more obsessed with sucking than others. Dummies can help you over this patch. If you don't like them, remember that you will be able to throw the dummy away as soon as the strong sucking need abates. There is no need for it to become a lasting habit.

- Adapt her sleep position. Babies who like to be held with some pressure on their tummies are often happier sleeping in a similar position. Current advice is not to put your baby face down to sleep. But you can swaddle her so that her tummy is firmly wrapped, then lie her on her side. Or use one of the special supports now available, where the baby lies on her side between a pair of mini bolsters.

• LEARNING TO GO TO SLEEP •

'My first baby never seemed to sleep,' says Chris, whose second baby is, at three months, an excellent sleeper. 'But it was my fault. I never trusted him to make it through the night. I constantly checked on him, and woke him up. He must have picked up my feeling that it wasn't safe to sleep. I always thought he would die. With this one, I feel she'll let me know if she needs me. I leave her to sleep in peace and she does.'

Learning to trust your baby to sleep, safe and sound, is part of the process of handing control of her sleep over to your baby. Even in these early weeks you can show your baby that sleep is something she can do for herself. This, together with the hunger cry and the core night, is the key to establishing sound sleep habits from the start.

But it can be difficult to trust your baby to sleep. Our increased awareness of cot death, in particular, can cause extra anxiety. Instead of gratefully relaxing when your baby is asleep, you may find yourself worrying about her.

• ANXIETY OVER A SLEEPING BABY •

Chapters 2 and 3 discussed parents' anxieties and how to deal with them separately from your baby. It's also a good idea to have your baby sleep in your bedroom so that you can see that she is all right and gradually get used to the idea that she can manage on her own. A carry cot or basket means a sleeping baby can be kept close, and taken into your room when you go to bed.

There is evidence that having your small baby sleep in the same room as you is a precaution against cot death. In societies where it's usual for the family to sleep together, cot death is unknown. Certainly the custom of putting a brand-new baby to sleep alone in a separate room with the door closed is unheard of in many countries, where some parents would consider it barbaric. It seems we will come to look back on this practice, which says more about Western affluence than about the needs of new babies, as a wrong turn. Sharing a room has real benefits for a new baby. Her immature breathing system may be stimulated by the breathing of others nearby, and their slight stirrings and rousings may help her establish her own sleep cycles. In this context it has been suggested that baby listening devices should ideally work the other way around. Instead of transmitting a baby's noises to her parents, a monitor should carry the sounds of her parents' breathing and sleeping to the baby. But there is no need for a baby monitor at all if your baby shares your room when she is very small.

• HANDING OVER CONTROL •

Letting your baby learn that sleep is something she can do for herself means letting her go to sleep on her own. She should be fed, winded, changed if necessary and then put into her cot or basket awake and relaxed. You might sit with her for a few minutes, singing a lullaby or gently patting her. Then you leave her to go to sleep on her own.

It sounds so simple. But some new babies strenuously resist being put down. You are just as likely to have a lively, irritable, muddled, new-born baby as you are to have an easy, placid, sleepy one. Making it sound easy is no help when it isn't. So when we say: 'Put her to bed and leave her to sleep,' it is a goal to aim at, not a foolproof recipe to follow.

Learning to go to sleep by herself is a crucial step for your baby. It shows her, from her earliest days, that sleep is something she can manage on her own. She finds she doesn't need a parent to 'put' her to sleep, and that's a big boost to her independence. And it means that, when she half-wakes, everything around her will be the same as it was when she went to sleep. To go back to sleep after reassuring herself that nothing has changed, she can simply repeat the way she went to sleep in the first place.

If, on the other hand, she gets the idea that she needs you to help her fall asleep, she will need your help to get back to sleep every time she stirs. So, from the very beginning, this is the golden rule: Let your baby go to sleep in bed on her own and, once she is asleep, disturb her as little as possible. When she does wake, and makes it clear she requires attention, keep it to a minimum. You want to meet her genuine needs, but you don't want to reward her for waking up. If you do, you will be programming her to wake for the reward of your company.

• NIGHT-TIME IS DIFFERENT •

At first your baby doesn't make a distinction between day and night. But that doesn't mean you shouldn't. The playful, cuddly feeds should be saved for the daytime. At night, feed and change your baby with no fuss and put her back to bed as soon as she is comfortable. Keep the lights low, and talk little and softly.

If she falls asleep while feeding or rocking, you may be tempted to wait until she is soundly asleep before you put her down. But you will, in the old phrase, be making a rod for your own back. The short-term benefit (no fussing at being put down) is not worth the long-term effects (your baby will cry when she half-wakes and finds herself in unfamiliar surroundings, and may soon be able to fall asleep only while feeding or rocking).

So don't hush the household, tiptoe to the cot, ease your baby in like a glass ornament and steal away. Lift her, change her if necessary, show her where she's going to sleep and let her be aware of being put into her bed. If she protests, give her a few minutes to settle and she is likely to fall asleep.

If she doesn't, try patting, singing and soothing words. If she seems to be winding herself up, rather than down, you may want to pick her up. But it's important that the day doesn't start all over again, because that cancels out your messages that it's time for sleep.

Your baby may need repeated settling at first. But she will soon get the hang of it. With this approach, progress is so rapid that your baby will start to sleep long stretches within a few weeks. It makes sense to use this early stage, while you and your baby are learning the ropes together, to encourage a sound sleep pattern. Once that's in place, your evenings will be your own and your sleep will be unbroken. And the earlier you start, the more you can take advantage of your baby's own biological tendency to adapt to sleeping all night.

One couple with a six-week-old son had never taken him out of his room after 6.30pm, no matter how many hours they had to spend in there soothing him. It seemed rather extreme, but it had worked. He had already accepted his 6.30pm bedtime and slept through the night. Not many parents are that determined. Apart from anything else, it seems like a bit of a grim evening for you. My own approach was a compromise. When my baby was a few weeks old and couldn't settle to sleep in the evening, I would put her in her car seat carrier, where she enjoyed watching us have supper. She was accepted, but given minimal attention, and put to bed again after half an hour or so. And that worked too.

Some parents see the first months as a perfect time to take their baby out at night, because she is confined to her basket or carrier, needs nothing but the odd feed and nappy, and can sleep anywhere. Occasionally, of course, that's fine. But if you want to use the early weeks to encourage your baby to sleep through the night, nightly jaunts into the fresh air, followed by several changes of scene, noise and new faces, don't do much to create an atmosphere of calm bedtimes and peaceful sleep.

• THE CORE NIGHT •

In her first days, cut off from the constant supply of food in the womb, your baby can't go for more than a couple of hours without being disturbed by urgent hunger pains. Then her immature digestive system may rebel against the sudden intake of food and cause discomfort.

Very soon, however – much sooner than you may have expected – your baby will show you that she can manage for longer without food, especially at night. She will do this by sleeping a 'core night', a block of sleep at night longer than one she has ever slept before. Typically she will do this at about one month old.

The core night is central to this approach to infant sleep. The next chapter covers it, and how to respond to it, in full. It is mentioned here because, along with learning your baby's hunger cry and helping her learn to go to sleep on her own, looking out for the core night is one of the key things you can do to consolidate her sleep pattern in the first weeks of life.

Sleeping a core night is a turning point for your baby. If you miss this signal, and continue to jump to feed her whenever she wakes, you are inadvertently sending her a clear message that what we do at night is wake up, to enjoy some food and company. This is the exact opposite of the message you want to send. Not only that, but her own first steps on the path towards sleeping all night will be reversed, instead of reinforced, by your influence. If you miss her cues that she is learning to manage a bit more on her own, you undermine her confidence in her growing independence. It is as if you are telling her that sleep is too difficult for her to manage on her own.

• LAYING THE FOUNDATIONS •

A good night's sleep may seem a far-off goal in these early days. But the sooner you get an unbroken night's sleep, the better for you. And the earlier your baby gets the habit of sleeping all night, the more deeply entrenched it will be. She will have begun to sleep soundly while she is still forming her first impressions of the world and how it works. Because staying asleep will be normal for her, it is much less likely to occur to her to wake up and demand attention.

If your baby has always slept all night, she is programmed to do it. Later, when she discovers her will-power, or when teething or some other disturbance causes wakefulness, her habit of going to sleep and staying asleep will be so firmly set that it will override any temporary disruption. She will be able to deviate from her solid sleep pattern and instinctively return to it, like a homing pigeon, when the cause of the upheaval is resolved.

But if your baby has never developed a sustained habit of sleeping all night, she doesn't have a base to return to. She literally doesn't know where she is when it comes to sleep. She will still try to sleep at night, and sometimes do so for a week or two, giving her parents the illusion that their problems are over. Yet without an established habit, any disruption, such as illness, travel or moving house, is likely to throw the whole thing off course. Before you know it, you have a baby of a year old who has never learnt to sleep through the night. And then it is much more difficult to teach her than it is when she is a tiny, impressionable baby.

SLEEP PLAN FOR YOUR NEW BABY

▶ Learn to detect your baby's hunger cry. Confirm it with the rooting reflex.

▶ Don't offer a feed unless the hunger cry is present. Try other ways of helping your baby relax.

▶ Try to meet your baby's needs during the day, so that she is less likely to need you at night.

▶ Be on the lookout for the first time your baby sleeps a 'core night' – a block of sleep at night longer than she has slept before. This is the beginning of being able to sleep through the night.

▶ Put your baby to bed awake and aware of her surroundings. Don't rock or feed her to sleep. If she drops off while you are doing this, rouse her gently and let her see where she is going to sleep.

▶ Feed or re-settle your baby if she wakes in the night with as little disturbance as possible. Save the cuddly, playful feeds for the daytime.

▶ Don't do anything your baby could interpret as a reward for waking up in the middle of the night.

5

THE CORE NIGHT
A Turning Point

'He slept from 10pm to 4am when he was six weeks old. Looking back, I see what a breakthrough that was. At the time I didn't know what to do with it. I just carried on as before. But he didn't do it again.'

Mother of Robbie, aged seventeen months, who has never slept through the night.

THE CORE NIGHT is the secret weapon in this approach. If you recognize it and build on it, your baby will be well on the way to sleeping all night, and a sleep problem will never develop in the first place. It is your baby's signal that he is ready to sleep for longer periods at night, when his system has matured enough to allow him to manage without food for more than three or four hours. It is called the core night because it is the heart of your baby's own, inbuilt sleep programme.

For you the core night is the foundation on which to build your baby's nightly sleep. It is a moment to be seized with both hands. Your baby is giving you the opportunity to consolidate his sleep into long, night-time blocks, and to extend these rapidly into what will become a permanent habit of sleeping all night.

The reason that the core night is so successful as a method of encouraging a young baby to sleep through the night is that the signal comes *from the baby*. It is not something that you impose on him, supposedly for his own good, but merely bewildering him and provoking resentment. It is your baby's own idea. All you are doing is getting the message.

If you do miss the golden moment presented by the core night, all is not lost. All the other principles in this book will still work, and your baby will still learn to sleep through the night. But using the core night from the beginning makes it astonishingly easy.

• DON'T TEACH YOUR BABY TO CRY •

Some programmes designed to cure sleep problems involve a lot of crying – sometimes hours of it. This is very hard on loving, concerned parents, even when you believe you're doing what's best. It also seems very hard on a young baby, who has no idea what's expected of him (unlike an older child), and can't understand why his parents' comforting presence has been withdrawn, just when he is telling them he needs it most.

The other problem with these methods is that they may actually teach a baby to cry. If he wants your presence and crying repeatedly brings it (even if only for a minute each time), he gets the message that crying will produce what he wants. If his crying doesn't make you come, he may go on crying in the hope that it will, but there comes a point when he doesn't know what he's crying for any more. Crying can become a habit like anything else. If a young baby can get into the habit of sleeping all night, it seems reasonable to assume that he can also get into the habit of crying.

Some parents can tolerate crying better than others. It depends on what you believe your baby is feeling when he cries – basically whether you sense that he is all right despite the crying or not. Some parents feel anguish when their baby cries, especially when he is tiny. There are good reasons for this. It is actually important for a baby's survival that his cries should be unbearable for his mother, because it prompts her to respond to him with food and care.

I remember a failed attempt on one occasion to eat supper while my two-week-old baby cried in her basket. As tears dropped into my spaghetti, my family said sensible, rational things intended to reassure me: the baby was fine, I needed to eat and so on. It made no difference. I put down my fork and picked up my baby, and then I was happy, and so was she. Other meals were eaten with one hand, the baby in the crook of my left arm.

Although not responding to cries from the cot will eventually result in your baby going to sleep, it is a miserable experience for you and quite possibly for your baby. It is all too easy to imagine him falling asleep in exhausted despair. Call it maternal instinct, a primitive survival mechanism, parental anxiety, whatever you like. But the whole idea of 'leaving him to cry' is intolerable to many parents. If this is the alternative, it's no wonder so many small babies are cuddled and rocked and fed to sleep, whatever the baby books say. It is not much good telling parents to do things that run counter to their instincts. Loving parents naturally want to do whatever it takes to keep their baby content.

The irony is that the reward for all this concerned attention may well be a sleep problem. Methods that settled a new-born baby are often carried on to become habits in an older baby, who has learned exactly what to expect from his parents. But it does not have to be a choice between leaving your baby to cry and never leaving him in peace.

• THE MAGIC OF THE CORE NIGHT •

The magic of the core night approach is not just that it works, and earlier than many parents think they have any right to expect; it also avoids unnecessary crying. Your baby's needs are met, when he has them. When he needs to sleep, that message is received and reinforced. Instead of encouraging him to cry for his parents, this method gives him the confidence to manage more and more by himself.

So how does it work? As Chapter 4 explained, you should be on the lookout for the appearance of a core night within the first few weeks of your baby's life. Typically your baby will sleep his first core night when he is about a month old.

What happens is this. You may be accustomed to your new baby sleeping for periods of no longer than two hours at night, or, if you are lucky, as long as four or five. It is unlikely there will be any sort of pattern at first – he may sleep for two hours, then four, or wake every hour and a half for two nights, then sleep a whole evening. Don't try to detect any direction in a brand-new baby. When you sense that this earliest, most intense phase of adjustment is passing (your baby's feeding will be well established, and both of you will probably feel calmer and less at sea), start to expect to see your baby's first core night. Your baby of about one month old will suddenly sleep a block of time at night longer than he has ever slept before.

For one restless baby, the first core night was five hours, from 10pm to 3am. With a more sleepy, placid baby, it might be six hours, perhaps from 7pm to 1am, or from 2am to 8am. (This last is so startling to parents accustomed to pre-dawn patrols that they may take half a day to recover from the shock to their system and completely overlook what it means to their baby.)

The point is not the number of hours, or what time of night they cover, but the fact that your baby has not slept that many before. (The first days of life do not count. Neither do daytime sleeps. Night-time sleep is your priority. The organization of daytime naps can come later.)

• LOOKING OUT FOR THE CORE • NIGHT

You may be thinking: 'This is all a bit vague. How can I be sure I'll know when my baby has slept a core night?' As an idea it may seem hard to pin down. But when it happens, you will know, if you are looking out for it. It makes a definite impression, even if you are unaware of its significance. Every parent I have talked to can remember a night when their small baby unexpectedly slept for longer than usual. Sometimes they look back on that night with a thoughtful expression, as if they are recognizing an opportunity missed.

'I WISH I had known about the core night when my baby was small,' says Harriet, whose son Robbie is a robust toddler who has never slept through the night for longer than a week or so. 'We went on holiday to France when he was six weeks old, and I remember how pleased I was when he slept for six unbroken hours one night. He had changed, but I didn't. I just carried on as before. I noticed it, but I missed it.'

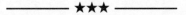

You might feel delighted when your baby first sleeps for longer at night, and assume he's got the hang of it. But be on your guard. Frequently a baby will wake after a much shorter time the next night. As you go to feed him, or pick him up, you might feel that what you had was a mere flash in the pan, and now you are back to square one. Perhaps he's not ready after all.

But he is. He just needs your help to consolidate what he has begun.

• TIME FOR ACTION •

There is a plan of action to follow, the minute you notice a core night:

- The key is to treat these hours as *your baby's night's sleep*, whenever in the night they happen to fall. They are the hours he has chosen for his first steps towards being able to sleep all night. In a way, he is experimenting with how it feels and to see if it's safe. You want to send back an encouraging, reassuring response. You do this by not interrupting his 'protected hours'.

- *Never feed your baby again during the hours that he slept through* in the course of his core night. He has shown you quite clearly that he can manage for those hours without food. Believe him.

- The next night, if he wakes during those hours, leave him alone for a few minutes to go back to sleep. He may not be sure if he wants anything or not, and he will probably go back to sleep in a short while. (Think of how we ourselves do this, if we wake in the middle of the night, while wondering if we should get up for a glass of water.) Many parents recall waking to a cry from their baby and falling asleep again while gathering the energy to go to him. They wake again later and are surprised to find that the baby has gone back to sleep on his own. They thought he needed feeding. But he is showing them that he has learnt to separate food and sleep. Freed from the urgent demands of his immature stomach, he is beginning to manage his own sleep process.

● If your baby does start serious crying during the hours of his core night, use other methods of settling him. If you pat and stroke him in his bed, it reinforces the message that it's still night-time and he should go back to sleep. If you pick him up, he's likely to become stimulated and more awake and will probably expect to be fed. If you do give him a cuddle, put him back down again when he is calm, so that he can go to sleep on his own.

● The goal is to disturb him as little as possible during his core night, to allow him to consolidate the longer sleeping pattern he has begun. Pat him, talk softly, hum a lullaby, tuck him in, offer a dummy or a sip of water. Do the minimum, while still reassuring him that you are there, all is well and it's time for sleep. He has already shown you that this is a time of night he can spend asleep. You are just reminding him of it.

● Remember that he takes his ideas about the world from you. Although his own body is adapted to being able gradually to sleep all night, impressions he receives from you can interfere with that programme. Try to convey an atmosphere of peace, quiet, calm and sleep.

If you follow this approach, within days your baby will sleep at least the hours of his core night every night. Now, although of course his night is still short compared to what it will be later, he has already learnt the most important of all sleep skills: how to go to sleep, and how to go back to sleep after surfacing. And he has learned all this while just a few weeks old.

His night may be short, but it is a real night, not just naps between feeds over the whole twenty-four hours. And that is the big difference between a new-born baby and one, just a few weeks older, who has begun to sleep a core night.

• BUILDING ON THE CORE NIGHT •

As soon as your baby is sleeping a core night, you can start to extend it. The most common time for a baby to choose to begin sleeping a core night is from about 10pm onwards. If your baby sleeps these hours at first, you will need to extend his core night backwards, towards the time you have chosen for his bedtime, as well as forwards, towards morning. Working backwards towards bedtime, put your baby to bed a bit earlier every night. Say to him: 'Now that you are getting so good at sleeping at night, I know you can sleep a bit longer.' This is to bolster your own confidence. Babies seem to adjust rapidly and easily. Your own doubts are far more likely to slow things down.

If your baby is one of those amenable sorts who starts to sleep his core night from the time that will become his bedtime, say 7pm, you need only work on extending his night's sleep towards morning. It is unusual for a baby to sleep a core night from the small hours of the morning until late: for example, from 4am until 9 or 10, but it does happen. If your baby chooses these hours for his core night, don't wake him earlier unless you have to. Just work on putting him to bed earlier and the late morning will adjust itself in time.

★★★

EIGHT weeks elapsed between my daughter sleeping her first core night, at four weeks, and establishing her permanent pattern of sleeping from 7pm to 7am. At first, I inched her bedtime forward by ten or fifteen minutes every few days. Then, as my confidence grew, I did it in leaps of half an hour at a time. She readily accepted every jump towards an earlier bedtime that I introduced and slept for a correspondingly longer time towards morning. With hindsight I could have done it faster.

As just one example of how smoothly the core night approach can work, here is a chart of our progress:

Age in weeks	Sleep starts	Sleep ends
4	10.00pm	3.00am
5	9.45pm	3.30am
6	9.30pm	4.00am
7	9.15pm	5.00am
8	9.00pm	5.30am
9	8.30pm	6.00am
10	8.00pm	6.30am
11	7.30pm	6.45am
12	7.00pm	7.00am

★★★

The advantages of this system are many:

- It follows your baby's lead.

- It is close to his own natural rhythms of sleep and waking.

- It helps him to separate sleep from food.

- It means no crying.

- It allows your baby to begin sleeping all night as soon as he is physically capable of it.

- It helps him begin to learn how to go back to sleep by himself if he wakes in the night.

- It works just as well with breast-fed babies as with bottle-fed ones.

This last point is of special interest.

• STARTING TO SEPARATE FOOD • AND SLEEP

It's commonly believed that breast-fed babies can't sleep through the night as early, or for as long, as bottle-fed ones. Because breast milk is more digestible, hunger is supposed to wake the baby sooner. But new research confirms many parents' experience: breast-fed babies, given the same ideal conditions for sleep as bottle-fed ones, show exactly the same good sleep patterns. Clearly, babies can separate their need for sleep from their need for food from very early on.

There is a school of thought that states you should wake your baby for a feed when you go to bed, to make him sleep through until morning. When mine was sleeping from 8.30pm until 5.30am, I tried it once. To my horror she woke up crying four hours later – something she had not done for weeks. I asked Lucy what I had done wrong.

'I could have told you she would do that,' she said. 'She woke early because you disturbed her natural sleep cycle by waking her at midnight, and a feed she hadn't been hungry enough to wake up for just confused her digestive system. She is finding her own rhythms of eating and sleeping, and the unecessary feed disrupted them.'

In Lucy's experience a baby woken for a feed at his parents' bedtime will often wake at the time he would have woken anyway, without the feed. If he does sleep through until morning, it's likely he could do that without the feed. For me it was a good lesson. It showed quite clearly that even a young baby has already begun to establish sleep cycles independent of his need for food. Sometimes there are medical reasons why a baby needs to be woken for feeds. But, for healthy, full-term infants who are gaining weight, this is Lucy's golden rule: Never wake a sleeping baby.

The relationship between food and sleep is discussed in full in the next chapter. The point here is how quickly your baby adapts and develops. While your new-born baby is a slave to his stomach and can't stay asleep when it's empty, by the time he is just a few weeks older, his nervous system and his digestive system have matured enough to allow him to go to sleep alone and content, and to stay asleep all night.

The core night is the key. It lets you follow your baby's lead, while at the same time making rapid progress towards a good night's sleep for him, and for you.

SLEEP PLAN FOR THE CORE NIGHT

▶ The core night is the heart of your baby's own, inbuilt sleep programme. It is the signal that he is ready to manage without food for long periods at night.

▶ Typically it will appear when your baby is about one month old. He will suddenly sleep for a longer stretch of time than he has before.

▶ The point is not the number of hours, or the time of night they cover. It is the breakthrough, for your particular baby, into a new, longer stretch of sleep.

▶ From the first time he sleeps a core night, never feed your baby again during those hours.

▶ Treat the core night as 'protected hours'. Think of it as your baby's night's sleep, although it will become much longer. At this stage it's quality, not quantity.

▶ Try not to disturb your baby at all during these hours. If he does wake, give him a chance to go back to sleep on his own.

▶ If he does need you to help him go back to sleep, reassure and settle him while keeping your intervention to a minimum. You don't want to give him the idea that sleep time is over.

▶ Start to extend his night by moving his bedtime closer to the time you have decided it will be, and/or encouraging him to go back to sleep if he wakes before the end of his core night. He will start to go to sleep earlier, and/or sleep later, as his ability to sleep for longer periods at night develops.

▶ Unless there are medical reasons that make it necessary for it, never wake a sleeping baby.

6

FOOD AND SLEEP
A Changing Relationship

'She snacks and naps. She sleeps in the evening, but wakes up several times after midnight and wants a bottle every time. She goes back to sleep after feeding, so she must wake because she's hungry. She probably needs the milk because she eats so badly during the day.'

Mother of Bethany, nearly one.

THE FEEDING relationship with a small baby is an intense one. When she is hungry, she cries frantically. Offered a feed, she stops crying at once. Her parents feel deep relief and gratification. They know they are doing something right.

From there, it's a small step to think of feeding as the essence of being a good parent. Women, especially, often experience food and caring as almost the same thing. Feeding *is* mothering. Mothering is feeding. Food is the answer, whatever the question. But even a new-born baby needs food only when food is what she needs.

Chapter 4 showed how important it is to learn to recognize your baby's hunger cry. It means you can feed her when she's hungry and find other ways of soothing her when she's not. It's also the first step in building communication with your baby, making it less likely that the two of you will run into misunderstandings and confusion.

• FEEDING CONFUSION •

If you feed your baby as soon as she cries, this is what can happen. Baby wakes up. Bewildered, she cries a little. Thinks: 'Am I hungry? I might be a bit peckish. I'm not sure. I'm confused. [Cries some more.] Oh, here comes a feed. Goody. I'll have that, then. Mmmm. Very nice. I feel all drowsy. I might just go back to sleep ... Hang on! What's this? I'm being put down. But I'm still hungry. Or sleepy. Or something. I don't know what I am!' [Cries harder than ever.]

This might seem fanciful, but it happens all the time. It happened to me. We got into a hopeless muddle. I rang the breast-feeding organizations for help, and they went on and on about 'the latch'. It made me feel as if I was some sort of apprentice locksmith. I wouldn't have minded, except that the latch (how the baby's mouth attaches to the breast) was perfect. The community midwife sat there saying so, and it matched all the diagrams in the books. And the breast-feeding counsellors didn't seem to want to talk about anything else. It got so bad that I dreaded asking anybody else for advice, in case they started talking about 'the latch'.

Then along came Lucy.

'That baby,' she said confidently, 'is the laziest feeder I have ever seen.'

I felt better at once. Suddenly it wasn't all my fault. I no longer felt like a failure as a nursing mother. My worry evaporated. I felt full of good will towards my lazy baby and eager to help her improve. Of course, it really meant a steep learning curve for me. I was doing lots of things wrong, but Lucy tactfully presented it from the baby's point of view.

'She doesn't feed properly, because she's not really hungry. If she had proper feeds, and her tummy got properly empty in between, she would be able to relax until she was genuinely hungry again, and sleep when she needed to.'

We began to untangle the muddle. These were the guidelines:

- Feed only when your baby is truly hungry. Confirm the hunger cry with the rooting reflex (see Chapter 4).

● Feed only for as long as your baby is feeding properly. Lucy calls this 'munching'. It is obvious that the baby is working hard. You can see her jaw moving as she swallows. Her ears may waggle, or her forehead go up and down.

● As your baby slows down and stops now and then, allow a few minutes of 'comfort sucking'. It's a bit like the end of a good dinner. A few chocolates or grapes make it perfect, but it's an extra, not part of the meal itself.

● Too much comfort sucking will make your baby over-full. That causes discomfort. Indigestion and hunger pains probably feel very much the same to your baby, so her cry may sound the same. You may think she's still hungry and feed her again. She may accept it, because sucking helps ease the discomfort. But the extra food will only make it worse.

● Don't allow your baby to fall asleep at the breast. You want her relaxed, full, ready to bring up any wind and perhaps be changed before she is settled for a sleep.

● If she does drop off, sit her up and get her to concentrate again before continuing the feed. Keep her at it by chucking her chin, or tickling her toes.

● Concentrate on the feed yourself.

● A baby who's feeding well will take up to ninety per cent of her feed in the first three minutes. Up to the end of the first month, when you and your baby are still learning the ropes, the whole business of feeding, winding and changing should still take less than an hour.

● It is *how* your baby feeds, the quality of the feed, that counts; not how long she spends at the breast, or how much she takes of her bottle.

● Some parents judge a feed a success if their baby falls asleep, because it proves she's satisfied and content. But she hasn't experienced the end of the feed or the transition to sleep, so she's not aware of how it feels to relax and go to sleep. Ideally she should end up with her eyes open, but glazed, in a sort of milk coma: 'looking drunk', as Lucy calls it.

• SLEEP CONFUSION •

It sounds like a lot of fuss over something that should be easy and natural. But it's all too easy to programme your baby to wake for food she doesn't need, or to make her unable to fall asleep except while feeding. Often it's the most concerned, loving parents whose baby can't sleep at night. They have been too quick to feed her, and, without meaning to, they have established firm ties between food and sleep.

Your baby is learning how to eat, and learning how to sleep. If what she learns is that we always eat until we fall asleep, that will become the only way she knows how to go to sleep.

Remember that everyone, babies, children and adults, wakes several times a night. A half-conscious check on our surroundings reassures us that everything is all right, and we turn over and go back to sleep. But when a baby who habitually falls asleep feeding stirs in the night, she finds everything all wrong. She is alone in her cot and the breast or bottle has disappeared. She startles into full alertness. Then, when she wants to go back to sleep, she can't, until the breast or bottle returns to establish the conditions she associates with falling asleep.

It is not that she is hungry. It is that she has not learnt how to go to sleep without feeding. While being helped to go to sleep easily, she has been given the wrong 'cues' for going to sleep. Instead of associating sleep with being in bed by herself in a quiet, darkened room, she associates it with feeding.

If she continues to feed regularly at night, she may even start to feel hungry at these times. This is learned hunger. We all become programmed to eat at certain times of day – our stomachs will 'tell' us it's lunchtime. Your baby will feel hungry in the middle of the night because that's when she's accustomed to eating.

These wrong sleep cues can grow up around all sorts of habits, such as rocking or walking a baby to sleep, until she can't go to back to sleep if she wakes in the night without being rocked or walked. But feeding is the most common cause of night wakings in babies under one year old.

★★★

WHEN Bethany was nearly a year old, Bryony had got night feedings down to a fine art. She lined up the bottles before she went to bed. Beth would wake, cry, be handed a bottle and go back to sleep. This happened two or three times a night.

Because she wanted only the bottle and required no attention from her parents, Bryony was convinced Beth was waking from hunger. During the day Beth ate poorly, and often seemed irritable. Bryony thought that if Beth ate more during the day, hunger might not wake her at night. So mealtimes became a battle between Bryony's persuasion tactics and Beth's resistance.

As Beth approached her first birthday, the whole family was getting fed up with the situation. Lucy's advice was asked.

'She's not waking at night because she's hungry,' she said. 'She's actually never hungry. She's eating poorly during the day because she's drinking so much milk at night. She just has a night feeding habit.

'She thinks you expect her to wake for her bottle. And, because she has always gone to sleep while feeding, she doesn't know any other way. When she half-wakes at night, as everybody does, she wants to go straight back to sleep. But she can't, because her cue for going to sleep is the bottle. When she gets it, she can go back to sleep.

'She's bad tempered and out of sorts during the day because she hasn't had enough sleep. That's how broken nights affect everybody.'

Bryony could have gone cold turkey and just stopped the night feeds. But she felt that Beth's protests would have been extreme and everyone's sleep would suffer even more. So Lucy suggested an alternative.

'Dilute her bottle with water,' she said. 'At first, make it a quarter water. Then, after a day or two, half water. Then three quarters, until it is all water. Beth will quickly decide for herself that she can't be bothered to wake up for water. Remember, she is tired, not hungry, and really wants to sleep all night. That's what her system needs.'

It worked in less than a week. Beth slept all night and woke hungry for breakfast. Her appetite and general mood improved out of all recognition.

'She's a really nice person now,' declared her grateful father. He too had assumed that Beth needed the night feeds and described the decision to stop them as 'counter-intuitive'.

★★★

• EVERYONE EXPECTS YOU TO FEED •
A CRYING BABY

Beth's father's genuine surprise that the answer was to feed Beth *less*, not more, reflects a common belief that a baby who wakes in the night must need feeding. Although continuing to offer feeds at night beyond when your baby needs them will prevent her from consolidating her sleep into a long, unbroken stretch, and from that point of view it is a mistake, parents can hardly be blamed for doing it.

Everyone seems to expect you to feed a crying baby. Grand-mothers, experienced mothers, doctors, midwives and health visitors all frequently assume crying, especially at night, is from hunger. No wonder parents come to believe it is 'intuitive' to respond to a cry in the night with food. Even when you know that the cry is not a true hunger cry, it is very difficult, under this kind of pressure, not to feed your baby. It is just easier than trying to sort out the underlying cause, especially when you are chron-ically short of sleep yourself.

Some breast-feeding mothers worry that their milk supply will suffer if they go for twelve hours without feeding at night. But your body adapts very quickly. Within days it will adjust your milk supply to fit the new feeding pattern.

Of course, if you are breast feeding, and want to stop feeding at night, you won't be able to use the watering-down method that worked for Beth. It is better to stop altogether, as giving just a little could make your baby furious. A half-way step, if night feeds have been long and playful, is to cut down to just a business-like feed, with the minimum of disturbance. When you do stop feeding, you could try giving a drink of water instead.

But if you follow the approach described in this book from the start, a night feeding habit will never develop in the first place. Night feeds will simply stop naturally when your baby is physically able to sleep through the night.

ONE-YEAR-OLD Joe's parents found a way of avoiding being disturbed by his early-morning awakenings. They put a bottle of milk in his cot when they went to bed. When Joe woke at 5am, he could just grab his bottle, drink it and go back to sleep. This allowed his parents to sleep, but it did nothing to help Joe learn to sleep later in the morning. He had good reason to wake at 5am, for the 'reward' of the waiting bottle.

It also meant that his system was tackling food at a time when it should have been at rest, so the quality of his sleep in the early morning was poor. The sleep after the bottle was more like a morning nap than part of a proper, unbroken night.

★★★

As a rule, never give your baby a bottle to take with her to bed.

- There is sugar in milk, and a lot more in fruit juice, and nothing could be worse for your baby's developing teeth than to bathe her mouth in sugar.

- Never having a bottle to hold when she's in bed by herself means your baby won't develop a habit of feeding herself to sleep. This 'wrong sleep cue' will make her unable to fall asleep without the bottle.

- If your baby always has her feed in your arms, you can keep an eye on how well she is feeding, as a guide to whether she really needs that feed or not.

This last piece of advice is especially useful at night. Make a point of noticing *how* she is feeding: Hungrily? Sleepily? Restlessly? Indifferently? When Lucy suggests looking out for this, parents often notice the night feeds are quite poor. That encourages them to try not feeding their baby at night, instead of jumping up at the first cry. They are frequently amazed to find their baby goes back to sleep by herself. A great leap forward has been achieved, simply by doing nothing. Doing nothing was, in fact, the appropriate response to the signals the baby was sending that she didn't really need that feed.

• GOING ALL NIGHT WITHOUT • FOOD

At about one month old, your baby's digestive system matures enough to allow her to start to separate sleep from food. She tells you when this has happened by sleeping a core night. After that, as Chapter 5 explained, she should not be fed during those hours.

Now your baby is sleeping for five or six hours at night without a feed, although she may still feed very frequently during the day. It takes up to a month for babies and parents to get the hang of the feeding process, and to master the communication that goes with it. While you are all learning, some babies may have as many as eight feeds over the twenty-four hours. But this quickly settles at about six.

If a baby of six weeks old is sleeping for eight hours at night, that leaves only sixteen hours for all her feeds. If she is still taking six feeds a day, you can see they will need to be quite close together. That doesn't matter. Sleeping all night is a big leap forward in her development and she needs whatever helps her to do it.

Many babies who sleep long hours at night from an early age seem to want a 'double feed' before their long sleep. It's as if they need to stoke up for the night. They give every sign of hunger just an hour or so after their early evening feed. It helps to be on the lookout for this, or you may find yourself thinking: 'She can't be hungry', while she loudly insists she *is*. It should be two separate feeds, even if they are close together, and not allowed to drag out into feeding all evening.

• FEEDING ON SCHEDULE •

It's commonly believed that bottle-fed babies sleep through the night sooner than breast-fed ones, because formula milk is less digestible and stays longer in the stomach. This is a factor that, understandably, convinces some mothers to bottle feed. But research now confirms that there is no difference in the age at which a breast-fed baby will sleep through the night, or for how many hours. How your baby's sleep is handled is much more important.

Breast-fed babies may well need feeding more frequently *at first*. But it doesn't follow that they are unable to sleep through the night as soon. By the time a baby is ready to start sleeping for long stretches, she is no longer a slave to her stomach. Remember that your baby is learning to separate food and sleep from the time she first sleeps a core night, at around one month old.

On scheduled feeding, feeds are gradually dropped until the baby is sleeping through the night. A new baby will have six feeds a day, one every four hours. The 2am feed is the first to go, after four to six weeks. Now the baby is sleeping from after her 10pm feed until an early morning feed at 6am. This is known as 'sleeping through the night', although it is, in fact, only eight hours – probably seven when you include the time the feed takes at night and waking before the feed is due in the morning.

Next to go is the 10pm feed. This frees your evening, and gives you a baby who sleeps roughly twelve hours a night – in this case, from after the 6pm feed until 6am.

Notice that dropping the 2am feed corresponds, in age, in approximately the number of hours actually slept, and even, in most cases, the time of night, to the core night that the baby will sleep of her own accord. Dropping the 10pm feed corresponds to extending the baby's night-time sleep, from the original core night to the bedtime you have chosen, and forward towards morning.

There is, in fact, very little difference in the actual sleep behaviour of the baby. The dropping-feeds approach looks simpler on paper, but it doesn't allow for a baby who doesn't fit this particular schedule, and it doesn't tell you what to do if your baby doesn't settle after her feed. As every new parent finds out, what looks simple on paper bears no resemblance to real life with a baby.

• DEMAND FEEDING •

Nowadays feeding on a strict, four-hourly schedule has, by and large, been replaced by feeding on demand. Clearly this is better for the majority of babies, whose body clocks are not set on a four-hourly cycle from day one.

- It means no miserable hours of crying for the baby, or listening to crying for you.

- It means you begin to communicate with your baby from the start, by learning the meaning of her different cries. This is how you both discover how she can tell you when she's hungry.

- It follows your baby's own rhythms, instead of unfairly imposing a timetable on a baby who can't tell the time.

Feeding on schedule did, however, have one advantage. It was good at getting babies to sleep through the night. It worked because, by the time the clock said you could feed her, you had, without any doubt, a hungry baby. Babies slept through the night as soon as they could (probably out of relief at not having to bawl for feeding, as much as anything else), and they were finished with night feeding before it stood a chance of becoming a habit.

Nothing makes the whole process of establishing regular rhythms of eating and sleeping run more smoothly than a baby who knows how to demand food when she's hungry, eat heartily and then relax into sleep. That's something we can learn from the success of schedule feeding in helping babies sleep through the night at an early age.

We rightly reject schedule feeding as cruel when it means leaving a hungry baby to cry ravenously, with no hope of satisfaction until the hands on the clock reach a certain position. But it is no kindness to a baby to feed her every time she opens her mouth either. At times it seems we have thrown the baby out with the clock. Demand feeding, which means feed your baby when she needs feeding, is now often taken to mean feed your baby whenever she cries, which does no good to anyone. Don't make her wait until the hands on the clock reach feeding time, but, just as importantly, don't feed her *before* she needs feeding either.

Imagine what it would be like if, every time you thought about food, a meal was placed before you. If you ate the food, because it was there, your stomach would protest, your body rhythms would be disrupted and your sleep would suffer. That's what happens when a baby is fed too often. It's doubly true when she is fed at night, when her digestive system and the rest of her body and brain should be resting, not dealing with feeds.

Like Beth, who was transformed into a happy baby with a hearty appetite for breakfast when she was given a chance to break her habit of waking to eat at night, your baby will clearly show you how glad she is to sleep all night, if you let her do it.

SLEEP PLAN FOR FOOD AND SLEEP

▶ Feed your baby only when she is really hungry.

▶ Feed her only as long as she is feeding properly and energetically.

▶ Allow a few minutes of comfort sucking, but don't prolong it indefinitely.

▶ Keep your baby concentrating on the feed, and concentrate yourself.

▶ Don't let her go to sleep while feeding. Regain her attention, and let her complete the feed awake but relaxed.

▶ Put her down before she goes to sleep.

▶ Keep night-time feeds short and to the point. Keep disturbance to a minimum.

▶ Never give your baby a bottle to take to bed with her.

▶ Concentrate on establishing a night's sleep without food, even if daytime feeds are still quite frequent. With your help your baby will adapt quickly to the different rhythms of day and night.

▶ Never feed your baby at night once she has begun to sleep through. Teething or other upsets will cause occasional broken nights, but offering a feed will only confuse the issue, and sow the seeds of a sleep problem. Use other ways of settling your restless baby.

▶ Remember that, given the right conditions, breast-fed babies can sleep through the night as early as bottle-fed ones. Your baby is able to start separating food from sleep from as young as one month old.

7

DAY INTO NIGHT
Habit and Routine

'Bed! Bed!'

Clementine, aged sixteen months.

WHAT HAPPENS at night is determined by what happens in the daytime. Just as our own sleep is affected by whatever is going on in our lives – stress, worry, lack of fresh air and exercise, and so on – it makes no sense to consider your baby's night-time behaviour in isolation from what goes on during his day.

This chapter deals with the time your baby is not supposed to be asleep. The next one discusses the normal disruptions that will inevitably occur, after his nightly sleep is well established, when he *is* supposed to be sleeping.

• USING THE FORCE OF HABIT •

We have seen how quickly habits can develop, even in quite young babies. Babies are strongly inclined towards repetition, because they are trying so hard to work out some rules for how the world works. From our own experience we know how powerful habits can be, and how difficult they can be to break. Habits grow out of the things we do every day. The way you care for your baby is your habitual way of doing things; the expectations this creates are the beginnings of his own habits.

Habit is a force that is always with us. Since we can't escape it, the best tactic is to use it. The idea is to encourage good habits and prevent bad ones from forming. Your best ally in this is routine.

Routine has rather fallen out of fashion. It came naturally when life was more orderly and predictable, and the pace was slower. It went with regular mealtimes, and plenty of time for domestic tasks and child care. Today life is complex, varied, flexible and often hectic. But this needn't mean routine is a lost cause.

To your baby, routine doesn't mean the exact time things happen. He can't tell the time. To him, it is to do with a series of cues, or signals, that he can come to depend on to tell him what happens next.

Babies show their pleasure in these sequences very early. A baby of just a few months old will react with delight to the sound of the key in the door which announces the return of a parent. For an older baby, lunch can become the event that is always followed by a nap – even if the time of the lunch, and of the nap, varies from day to day. And a baby is well programmed for sleep if it invariably follows as the next step in a 'dance' that goes: bath, supper, bed. It's the sequence that counts, not the precise time of day.

Babies feel secure when they know where they are, and what is going to happen next. So do some parents. Some of us set more store by the clock than others. I was devoted to the idea of a 7pm bedtime. Once it was in place, it was varied only for special occasions. My baby duly became as avid a clock watcher as I was. 'Bed! Bed!' she said, shown her cot on the dot of seven. As a baby, Lucy's daughter, Emma, would actually crawl towards her cot at bedtime.

I like it like that. Other parents might feel they were being dictated to by the clock. The point is it doesn't matter. You can decide what suits you. The routine is the thing, not the time, or doing it at exactly the same time every day.

All within reason, naturally. A morning nap may vary in time, and length, from day to day. But if it doesn't happen on a pretty regular basis, you can't expect your baby to stay in the habit.

• When to Introduce a Bedtime • Routine

A good time to introduce an evening routine is when your baby is about two months old. The earlier you start, the more deep-seated the bedtime habit will be; but two months is about as early as you can reasonably expect it to work. Before that he hasn't got enough of an idea of what going to bed is, never mind sleeping until it's time to get up, for it to mean much to him.

It may help to measure the first few months against Lucy's timetable:

- It takes about two weeks for you and your baby to adjust to his presence in the world. This is the extreme new-born stage. It can be rather harrowing for everybody, so it's best not to expect an idyll of domestic harmony. New parents are bombarded with rosy images of couples gazing down in united bliss at their infant. It is worth noticing that these babies are all about four months old.

- Over the second two weeks, confidence is built up. Your baby begins to trust that his needs will be met. You begin to adjust to being parents, if you are new parents, or to your new baby's place in the family, if not.

- Once this process is under way, usually by the time your baby is about a month old, he will begin to sleep a core night. This happens as a combination of the baby's maturing digestive and nervous systems, and the reduced anxiety level in him and his parents.

- The core night is a watershed. After it appears, your baby will progress quickly towards sleeping all night, given the right conditions, and if night-time feeding during his long sleep time is stopped. By three months, many babies are able to sleep for ten or twelve unbroken hours a night.

- His new ability to sleep for long stretches at night shows that your baby has begun to adjust to our rhythms of sleeping at night and eating during the daytime.

• This is a good time to introduce a bedtime routine, to consolidate the distinction between day and night, and to start cultivating a habit of going to bed. He may not have been formally put to bed until now. From now on he should be.

• BEDTIME •

Put your baby to bed. It may seem obvious, but it doesn't always happen. Babies who are allowed to stay up until they are exhausted, and fall asleep wherever they happen to be, are not being given good sleep habits. It leaves too much up to them. When they wake in the night, or in the early hours, they have to decide all over again: 'Where am I? Do I like it? Am I still sleepy? Should I wake up?'

Babies can't handle that much choice about something as fundamental to their well-being as sleep. If they are given the idea, from as early as they can begin to grasp it, that we go to bed at bedtime and stay there until morning, life is easier and pleasanter for them (and for you) than it is if they are left to make it up for themselves as they go along.

If you let a baby decide for himself when and how he needs to sleep, you can't be surprised if he makes a hash of it. He doesn't want the responsibility. It is more than he can handle, and it creates anxiety and confusion. He wants you to assure him that you are in charge, and he is all right. That leaves him free to get on with his own business of growing and learning – and sleep plays a large part in both.

Where Should Your Baby Sleep?

The benefits for a small baby of sleeping in the same room as his parents have already been mentioned. Some parents choose to have their baby in bed with them. There is one view that this is best for your baby. Certainly it can help to reassure an anxious new-born, and allow him to make a more gradual transition from life in the womb to his new, separate and increasingly independent existence.

Lucy's own view is that a baby is better off in his own bit of space from the start. In her experience both babies and parents sleep better in their own bed. In bed with you, your baby may wake more frequently and your presence may stimulate him to demand a feed he doesn't need. This could interfere with the development of his own regular sleep cycles. In turn, your baby's movements may wake you while he remains asleep – and you need sleep as much as he does.

A good compromise is to put your new baby's cradle or basket right next to your bed, so that you can pat him, talk to him and pick him up without having to get up yourself. It makes it easy to cuddle up with your baby when he needs physical contact, while still allowing him to learn that he has his own place to sleep.

When your baby is about two months old, and more settled and 'together', you could move his bed further away – perhaps to the foot of your bed or across the room. This move reflects and encourages your baby's growing ability to manage on his own. Exactly when you move your baby to a room of his own, or in with other children, will depend on your circumstances and your preference. Your baby gets the greatest benefits of sharing your room in the first three months.

There does come a time (often around the end of the first year) when, if you are still in one room, you and your baby start waking each other up. His sleep will be disturbed by your coming in and by your stirrings in your sleep, and you may be woken by his movements and noises. He is much more likely to demand your attention when he half-wakes, just because you are there, visible and available. At this stage, sleeping in your room is stimulating, rather than reassuring, for your baby, and he, and you, will sleep better if you can move him out.

Bathtime

The evening routine begins with a bath. If bathtime has been in the morning, as a fresh start after the events of the night, now is the time to switch it to the evening. A warm bath is relaxing, and works as a signal that bedtime is not far off.

One of the nicest and easiest ways to bathe a small baby is with you. Your baby feels securely held and that helps him relax.

As well as holding him close against your chest, lie him on his back, supporting his head and bottom. This encourages him to begin stretching and exercising his limbs. In the big bath, there is plenty of water to support his movements. There is no strain on your back, so you are more relaxed, and that means your baby is relaxed too.

Small babies are slippery, so this is best with someone to help. Ideally one of you gets in the bath and the other undresses the baby and hands him in, and afterwards takes him back and dries him. For a parent just coming home from work, this can be an immediate, warm and intimate way of getting involved in the baby's day.

Baby Massage

After the bath is the time to try some baby massage. This is especially useful for boosting your confidence if you sometimes feel a bit nervous handling your baby. Some jumpy babies are relaxed by being touched in a relaxed, deliberate way. There is also evidence that this type of patterned, skin-to-skin touching can help strengthen the immune system.

You need a warm room, warm hands and a warm baby. Start by relaxing your own shoulders and arms, and rub some oil (olive, vegetable, baby or almond) between your palms. Then stroke your baby gently, starting at the top of his head. Move downwards over his limbs, and out over his hands and feet. Stroke him clockwise on his tummy, in the direction of his digestive system.

Night Clothes

Now dress your baby in his night clothes. There has not been much point in these until now. New babies may need several changes of clothes, or none at all, over the twenty-four hours. But by the age of two months or so, your baby is likely to be out and about a bit more, and spending some time on the floor, so he will need something more than a sleepsuit or nightgown in the daytime. Soft, cuddly night clothes are soothing.

Quiet Time

Settle down for an especially close, quiet feed. Make this the baby's protected time, if you can. Babies adjust to anything, and the hubbub of family life may not seem to bother them. But try to take time out yourself, to give your baby a chance to relax with you before bed.

This is the time that you and he might spend together when he is older, chatting about his day. At this age you send the same reassuring message by being physically and emotionally close. Good sleep, for your baby, means separation without anxiety. You will be giving him a feeling of being loved and cared for that he will be able to carry with him into sleep.

Try to be calm and relaxed yourself. This is easier said than done. A baby's bedtime routine coincides with a busy time in most households – people are coming home, cooking has to be done, other children need attention, the telephone rings. There's a lot to distract both you and your baby.

Babies are often fretful at this time of day, just when you feel they should be winding down. They are tired, sometimes 'burnt out' and over-stimulated, sometimes just ignored and bored. Your baby will also cry if you are anxious. You are his security, so when he senses worry or distress in you, he feels under threat. If his fretfulness makes you tense, he will forget his original reason for crying and complain until he feels you, and he, are all right.

You may find yourself saying: 'I don't know what he wants.' What he wants is relaxed, amusing, happy parents, to make him smile, tell him all is well, he is loved and that it's time to go to sleep. In the real world what he often gets is tired, harrassed parents, who wish he would go to sleep so they can get on with everything else, or just have some much-needed time to themselves. But if you can carve out fifteen minutes of calm, it will be easier for your baby to go to sleep and stay asleep, and your evening will be your own.

Going to Bed

Show your baby where he is going to sleep. This lets him know where he will find himself when he stirs in the night, so he isn't surprised or frightened by unexpected surroundings. Make his basket or cot cosy and welcoming. You might want to show him his teddy bear or other soft toy, to encourage him gradually to come to see it as a friendly 'comfort object' to take to bed with him. But at this stage, fluffy toys don't mean much to him, so keep them to one or two. If he still likes being swaddled, wrap him firmly but leave his arms free. Tuck him in securely.

Texture is important to some babies, and smell to others. Some like warm, soft flannel sheets, others prefer crisp cotton. Some babies seem to be soothed by sleeping on a lambskin, first developed for use in premature baby units and now available in the shops. If you have one, it's a good idea to sleep on it yourself first, so that it smells of you.

If your baby seems restless, try changing his sleeping position. Some babies are happy only lying on their tummies. Current advice is not to put babies to sleep face down. So what do you do if yours can relax only when lying on his front?

- Try to give him the pressure on his tummy, and the feeling of being in contact, that he prefers.

- He may like being swaddled, wrapped firmly in a flannel sheet.

- Lie him on one side, supported by his underneath arm, with his tummy touching the mattress.

- A small pillow tucked against his tummy when he's lying on his side sometimes helps.

- There is a device on the market which consists of two mini bolsters joined by a strip of fabric. The baby lies on his side, supported between the bolsters.

Once your baby can roll over, he will find his own preferred sleeping position. Some babies like to feel their feet touching the bottom of the bed, others will work themselves up until their heads are touching the top. Follow what seems to be your baby's preference when putting him down.

You might want to sit with your baby for a few minutes, perhaps talking softly or singing, while he settles down. A musical toy that plays a lullaby can act as a substitute for your presence and help your baby let you go. Some babies are happy in the dark; others like the glow of a night light. Say 'good night' in a very positive way and leave the room.

Don't expect it to work at first. It sometimes takes a week or so before your baby is confident enough to go to sleep without a reassuring visit. If his protests last more than a few minutes, go through the settling and 'good night' routine again, leaving when he is calm. If he gets himself in a state, you may want to pick him up to soothe him. But don't feed him, take him out of the room or give him any idea that the day is starting over again. You are trying to let him discover that he can go to sleep by himself, and he won't learn it if he doesn't get the chance to try it out.

Once your baby is in the habit of going down easily at bedtime and sleeping until morning, you can congratulate yourself on your success. He is settled into a pattern that should form the basis of a lifetime's good sleep habits. Now your role is to try to make sure that nothing interferes with it.

As part of his normal growth and development, there will be times when your baby will wake in the night and be unable to fall asleep again without your help. He will also go through occasional bouts of resisting his bedtime. These episodes may last a couple of days or a few weeks. They are nothing to worry about, and there is no reason why these brief disruptions should lead to a sleep problem.

However, sometimes a baby is wakeful for a night or two for a good reason, and the response he receives encourages him to continue to wake at night, until it becomes a habit. The same is true of bedtime protests. The key to avoiding this is to understand the cause of the original disturbance, so that you can respond appropriately, and limit it to a minimum. This kind of wakefulness is the subject of the next chapter.

• DAYTIME NAPS •

We have concentrated on night-time sleep for two good reasons. One is that it is so essential for parents. The other is that a baby who sleeps well at night will thrive. His temper and appetite will be good, and the whole business of food and naps will be easier. A tired, irritable baby, whose broken nights are preventing his metabolism from settling into healthy rhythms, may be too tense to enjoy his meals and rest-times.

But although night sleep is the priority, daytime naps are important too. They give parents a much-needed break. And even a short sleep transforms a fretful, dissatisfied baby into a cheerful, enthusiastic one. Without naps your baby will become over-tired and reach a point of frantic exhaustion just when he should be ready for a relaxed winding down at bedtime.

For you, your baby's bedtime is the home stretch in a long day. But for him, the ritual of his bath and quiet feed and cuddle is a high point: pleasurable time spent basking in your full attention. He needs some reserves of energy left to enjoy it.

Some parents believe daytime naps will make a baby less ready to sleep at night. This is true only of babies over a year old. These older babies do best when they sleep somewhere around the middle of the day, as a late afternoon nap will indeed mean that they are not sleepy at bedtime. But for young babies, sleep is so central to their healthy growth and development, physical and mental, that it's almost true to say they can't have too much sleep. Sleeping is a habit, and the more babies sleep, the more they sleep.

In the early days, naps pretty much take care of themselves. A new baby just falls asleep when he is sleepy, unless something is preventing him. As your baby begins to consolidate his sleep into a long stretch at night, his naps will tend to fall into a natural pattern around that. A baby who sleeps well at night is likely to be rested, relaxed, happy and eating well, so he will find it easy to settle down for regular daytime naps.

A rule of thumb is that most babies need two naps a day, one in the morning and one in the afternoon, until they are about a year old. After that they usually drop one or the other, and the remaining nap settles at around the middle of the day. Some children keep this nap until they go to school, others drop it before they're three, or turn it into a rest with some books and toys to play with.

Your baby's naps will adapt to his changing need for sleep. The only thing that can make it difficult to stick to a regular nap time is when a baby wakes at widely different times in the mornings. If your baby gets up at 5am one day and 8am the next, he will have a lot of catching up on his sleep to do the first day, but feel wide awake the second. Any pattern is likely to go out of the window. This is one good reason to encourage regular hours at night. Daytime sleeps should be seen as additions to a long, unbroken night, not as substitutes for it.

Once naps settle into a pattern, their length will vary. One day your baby may sleep for half an hour, the next for three hours. Let him sleep, if possible. If he has to be woken to go out, let him think he has woken up naturally. Open the door quietly and potter nearby. Draw the curtains. When he wakes, welcome him gently. You will be encouraging him to think of sleep as something that begins and ends easily and pleasantly. If he is often startled awake and briskly roused, he may develop a habit of becoming instantly alert when he half-wakes, instead of remaining drowsy and drifting back to sleep.

Babies often sleep better in the fresh air. If your baby is well wrapped up, in a windproof pram, where you can see and hear him, he can have his daytime sleeps outside whenever it is not actually raining. Leaves moving overhead seem to have an almost hypnotically soothing effect. As he grows you will be able to watch your baby gurgle and wave when he wakes, and swipe at toys strung across his pram. Discovering he has his own resources for entertainment shows him he doesn't need to call for you as soon as he wakes.

• HOW MUCH SLEEP DOES A BABY • NEED?

Babies vary in the amount of sleep they need, as in everything else. Charts showing average amounts of sleep for babies of different ages only confirm how much variation there is. There is one simple, foolproof way to know if your baby is getting enough sleep: your baby has had enough sleep if he wakes up happy.

If he wakes grizzly and fretful at 5am, he is tired. He does not need to start the day. He will only stagger through it until he has a nap anyway. Re-settle him as if it were the middle of the night and explain that it's not time to get up yet. Even if he fusses and doesn't go back to sleep, it's worth hanging on until a time you could reasonably call morning – perhaps 6am. It all helps to give him the idea of staying in bed until it's time to get up.

On the other hand, if he wakes chuckling, gurgling and smiling at 5am he has, regrettably, had enough sleep. He may still be amenable to another hour or so in his cot, given some entertainment, and he may well sleep more when he is a little older. Try making his morning nap a bit later. This will separate his nap more completely from his night's sleep and encourage him to consolidate his night-time sleep into a longer single block. But waking happy is a sure sign that he has had enough sleep for this particular night or nap.

• How Can You Tell When Your • Baby Needs to Sleep?

The same rule applies in reverse when your baby is tired. So, just as you can tell when your baby has had enough sleep, because he wakes up happy, you can tell when he needs to sleep, because he becomes less happy. A small baby will fret and may cry miserably, quite a different sound from the lusty bawl of hunger. Rubbing his fists in his eyes is a sure sign of tiredness. Babies of all ages do this.

A bigger baby will, quite suddenly, change his behaviour. One minute he will be playing happily; the next he's clumsy, his concentration and enjoyment have evaporated, and he irritably discards one toy after another – he seems to disintegrate before your eyes, almost as if he is short-circuiting. This is the time to scoop him up and bear him off for a quiet time together, followed by a sleep.

When your baby wakes happy after his sleep, make a fuss of him. Show him how pleased you are to see him, and tell him he's wonderful. It's easy to take good sleep for granted, but in fact it's a considerable skill, and your baby deserves plenty of praise for mastering it.

SLEEP PLAN FOR GOOD HABITS AND ROUTINE

▶ Aim to encourage good habits and prevent bad ones.

▶ Remember that creating a consistent set of signals that lets your baby know what to expect is more important than the time on the clock.

▶ Introduce a bedtime routine after your baby has begun to sleep long stretches regularly at night. A good time is at about two months.

▶ Try to carve out some 'protected time' to give your baby an especially warm, close, calm feed before bed. It will give him a feeling of being loved and cared for to carry with him into sleep.

▶ Show your baby where he is going to sleep. Tuck him in, say good night in a positive way and leave the room.

▶ Don't expect it to work at once. Your baby may need time to get the hang of bedtime. Keep reassuring him, and keep your routines consistent.

▶ Watch your baby for signs of tiredness, and let him have a sleep when he shows fatigue. Don't let him become over-tired.

▶ Your baby has had enough sleep when he wakes up happy.

▶ When he wakes up, praise your baby for sleeping well and give him a big welcome.

8

GOOD NIGHTS, BAD NIGHTS
Why is my Baby Awake?

'I'm more than happy to help her get back to sleep when she's uncomfortable, because it happens so seldom. If she woke at night all the time, I wouldn't be able to think straight, and I would get fed up with her.'

Mother of Anna, eight months.

IF YOUR BABY is one of those naturally good sleepers who seems to sleep well with no help right from the start, perhaps you feel a lot of this book doesn't apply to you. But good sleepers can turn into bad sleepers, when something crops up that disturbs them. You will be able to help your baby through these patches by finding out the reason for the disruption, responding appropriately and encouraging her to return to her usual pattern before a sleep problem has a chance to develop.

Without this approach, parents of babies who usually sleep well may be thrown by a sudden run of broken nights. If your baby has never had any trouble sleeping at night, you may feel at a loss when she suddenly can't do it any more. If you're thinking: 'What on earth is going on?', your uncertainty is communicated to your baby, and this makes it more difficult for her to settle down again.

• HOW SLEEP PROBLEMS DEVELOP •

Sleep problems can crop up at any age. They happen when waking, for any reason, develops into regular waking, out of habit. They also happen when a problem that is causing a baby to wake is overlooked and so goes on persistently disturbing her sleep.

A sleep problem can creep up on you. The first night your baby is wakeful, you may put it down to a cold or a bad dream. Before you know it, it's happened every night for a week. The second week, you start wondering what's causing your baby to wake. By the end of a month, your baby has developed a habit of refusing to sleep, and a sleep problem is well under way. That's why it is so important to be on the lookout for causes of wakefulness, so as to try to sort them out at once and nip any problem in the bud.

As part of normal growth and development, every baby goes through episodes of waking and crying at night, and bouts of resisting bedtime. When it happens, don't panic. It doesn't mean you are about to lose everything you have gained. These disruptions should last no more than a week or two at most, and, with your help, they will not damage your baby's generally sound sleep pattern. The key is not to deviate from your usual night-time drill, beyond responding to your baby's specific needs. A wakeful episode does not change the basic rule that night-time is for sleeping.

• A SOUND SLEEP FOUNDATION •

It is enormously easier if your baby usually sleeps well. If the disruption appears as a marked deviation from a pattern of generally sound sleep, the problem shows up immediately, so you can deal with it as soon as possible. It also makes your baby as keen to resolve the problem as you are. She will be bothered by waking up and want to return to what feels familiar and normal. And that, for her, is sleeping all night.

If your baby has never slept well at night, her nights will also be disturbed by normal events like teething. But it is much harder to spot the new cause of her restlessness when it comes on top of an already muddled sleep pattern. And when you are suffering from chronic fatigue yourself, the clear thinking and the patience you need to sort out the problem are in short supply.

The whole question of sleep can dissolve into a blur of bewilderment and exhaustion, a tangle of bad habits and new problems that is impossible to unravel. It's no wonder that many parents give up, and decide to wait for their baby to grow out of it. The trouble is, she may not. Although the *causes* of waking may go away by themselves, the *habits* of bad sleep they lead to can be persistent. Half of all babies who have a sleep problem at one year old still have it at three.

This chapter suggests how to work out what is causing your baby to be wakeful and how to arrive at a solution appropriate for your particular baby. We will look first at causes of disturbed nights, then at the method for handling them.

• WHY THIS APPROACH WORKS •

This method allows you to continue building communication with your baby while she is going through a difficult patch and needs it most. It avoids applying a blanket solution to all sleepless babies, overlooking the vital differences of age, temperament and family circumstances.

Although sleep programmes that provide a 'recipe' for you to follow will cure some habits, they do nothing to help you and your baby learn to negotiate life's hurdles together, and get to know each other better by doing it. They also don't help you understand underlying problems that cause wakefulness. If anything, they sow the seeds of conflict and resentment, as they involve setting your will against your baby's. In any battle of wills, by the nature of things, you should certainly win. But sleep isn't a good arena for battles.

Waking up and crying is how your baby tells you something is preventing her from sleeping well. What she needs is to have her crying listened to and understood. Just feeling understood, by itself, will make a difference to how secure and relaxed she feels, and so help her to sleep.

Understanding her makes a difference to how you respond too. Sometimes it will mean simply reminding her that it is night-time and she needs to go to sleep. At other times she will need comforting, or some extra attention during the day. On the other hand, if she is angry, she could be infuriated by your efforts to console her, and you may have to let her express her feelings without intervening.

• WHY IS MY BABY AWAKE? •

The first step is to look for the reason why your baby has woken up, or can't get to sleep.

- Listen to your baby's cry and notice how she behaves. Try to work out how she is feeling. Tired? Miserable? Restless? Angry? Frightened?

- Notice her response when you go to her. Is she immediately comforted by seeing you? Does she want something (food or play) from you? Does your appearance make no difference, or seem to make her cry harder?

- Think about what is going on in the daytime. Have there been any changes in your baby's life? She may manage fine all day, but anything that is bothering her may surface at the vulnerable time of separating from her parents to go to sleep, or prevent her staying asleep.

- Look at her routine. Is she happy in the daytime? Does she seem settled in her feeding and sleeping? Is she getting fresh air and exercise?

- Consider what is happening in your own life. If you are depressed, worried or unhappy, this can disturb your baby's sleep. You may not be able to change your circumstances, but you can change the way your baby is affected.

- Look at the disturbance as something temporary, that you and your baby can solve together. Don't blame your baby or yourself.

Three things will cause periods of wakefulness in virtually all babies, no matter how settled their usual sleep pattern. They are teething, developmental spurts and anxiety.

• TEETHING •

Teething, like colic (which is discussed in the next chapter), is difficult to get a handle on. Some people believe both complaints are little more than convenient explanations for behaviour which may have more complex causes. Certainly teething does not make babies ill. On the other hand there is a definite range of specific symptoms associated with teething, some of which can cause discomfort severe enough to wake a baby in the night.

The first tooth often causes trouble, and so do the first molars. Some time between four and eight months, your baby may wake and cry in the night. She may go off her food, have a bout of diarrhoea, be hot and bothered, display one bright red cheek, dribble, constantly put her fist in her mouth, or be generally fretful and miserable. This is teething, and it can happen off and on for the first two years.

Symptoms need not immediately be followed by a tooth. It's the stirrings of the teeth as they make their way to the surface that's troublesome. The actual cutting of the tooth may go unnoticed. But teething in general, accompanied by one or more of the symptoms described, is a classic cause of disturbed sleep in babies under two.

There is not a great deal you can do to help a teething baby sleep, except offer her your sympathy and understanding. There are various gels and drops on the market designed to calm inflammation of the gums. Chamomilla granules, a homeopathic remedy, have a soothing effect. If your baby is hot, you may want to give her infant paracetamol to bring down her temperature.

• DEVELOPMENTAL SPURTS •

There will also be disturbances in your baby's sleep as she goes through the various stages of her development. Developmental spurts commonly occur at roughly the following ages, often accompanied by specific changes in behaviour:

- **Six weeks**: marked development in the central nervous system and shifts in brain activity. Unexplained crying may be related to this. Your baby is becoming able to hold her head up: control over her body starts from the top. Her new ability to exchange smiles means lots of social interaction. She will spend longer periods awake to enjoy this.

- **Three months**: consolidation of maturity in brain processes. This may cause another phase of unexplained crying. Now she can control her shoulders and play with her hands, using them to explore people and objects. She looks at toys and delights in accidentally making them move or rattle. She is taking in massive amounts of information from her environment. Her waking time now has definite play periods.

- **Six months**: your baby will be eating solids and may be starting to sit up. She may achieve mobility by rolling across the floor to reach desired objects. This shift is usually a positive, exciting one, but new abilities may cause some anxiety. It's also a common time for teething trouble.

- **Nine months**: a major landmark. At about this age your baby develops the ability to keep herself awake at will, so disturbances of her sleep may be more troublesome, as she can now stay awake even if exhausted. Starting to crawl may be a breakthrough that helps her sleep better after the frustrations of immobility, or it may make her anxious about being out of sight of her parents. The enormous expansion of her understanding of herself as a separate individual may make a normally easy-going, friendly baby suddenly anxious, clingy and suspicious of strangers. Separation at bedtime may be a problem at this stage.

- **Approaching one year**: her will-power becomes strong as she prepares to assert her independence, the major effort of the toddler years. This may lead to furious protests at bedtime. She is finding her feet. New-found walking skills may happily resolve a period of frustration. Sometimes, though, her increasing independence worries her, and anxiety will show up in her sleep behaviour.

It helps to be on the lookout for these shifts in your baby's development. You will be more prepared for bouts of wakefulness, so more able to understand them and reassure your baby in a way that will help her get back to her normal sleep pattern as soon as possible.

• ANXIETY •

Anxiety is not a word we naturally associate with babies, whose lives seem carefree compared with our own. But the barrage of new information they must continually process, the constant stream of new experiences, and the conflict of depending completely on you while becoming aware of themselves as separate individuals, all add up to considerable stress.

Babies are adapted to this steep learning curve and usually they cope well. But sometimes a big event or a change in their lives, even a change in a parent's mood, can tip them over the edge, as it were, and they experience a kind of stress overload. It is very likely that their sleep will be disturbed, because they need to feel safe, secure and protected if they are to separate happily from their parents and stay asleep all night.

We have looked at the range of new anxieties that can go with your baby's developing independence and abilities. We could say these stresses come from inside the baby, while the kind we are discussing now come from outside.

Below are some typical examples of the kind of events that can lead to disturbed sleep. You will be able to think of many others, relevant to your own family circumstances. It's worth remembering that the disturbance need not be directly tied to the event itself. Sometimes your baby will seem to take a big change in her stride. Then, perhaps prompted by her feelings as she thinks through what has happened, she may react a week or two later with a patch of disturbed sleep.

- Moving her bed, perhaps out of her parents' room into a room of her own.

- Moving house.

- A change in her child care arrangements.

- A change in her routine.

- Starting solid food.

- Giving up the breast or bottle.

- Mother going back to work.

- The birth of a sibling.

- Parents being distressed by something in their own lives.

- Travel.

- Even thrilling experiences, like Christmas or a day at the zoo, may over-stimulate your baby and make her sleep less well.

• How to Handle Bad Nights •

Your response will naturally vary according to the kind of disturbance your baby is showing and what you believe may be the cause. There will be times when there is nothing you can do to change things, and your baby just needs time. When this happens, don't feel you can't help. Just showing that you understand her feelings and the reasons for them will make a big difference to your baby's feelings of confidence and security, and so help her to return to a sound sleep pattern.

Reassurance

You could say to her, for example: 'I know you feel upset, because we're in a new house, and everything seems different and strange. But don't worry. I am here to look after you, you are completely safe and everything is all right. It's night-time now, time to go to sleep.'

You might have to go through this routine several times a night for a week or so, until your baby settles down. It might take just a night or two. It can seem tedious and frustrating. But the very fact that you constantly repeat this message, and that your behaviour is consistent in a changing world, reassures your baby and helps her to sleep.

The same applies when something is wrong in your own life, perhaps making you upset, depressed or unusually anxious yourself. Just being aware of your own feelings will help you deal with them and make it less likely that your baby will be disturbed.

Your baby will be less bothered by the expression of feelings (crying or the odd outbreak of shouting are, after all, within her own range of experience) than she will be by underlying tension, which affects your relationship with her. Tension is caused by feelings which have not been recognized or expressed. It can come as a great relief to your baby, as well as to you, when the air is cleared.

If your baby does seem difficult when you have problems of your own, it can help to make a point of reassuring her that everything is all right. Don't imagine she doesn't notice anything amiss. Remember that you are her security; she will worry if she senses conflict in you.

Daytime Answers

Sometimes there is more specific action you can take, but you may have to do some lateral thinking to find it. It's easy to fall into ways of handling your baby that make the problem worse. You might think, for example: 'She's probably waking to see me at night because I have gone back to work and she feels she isn't getting enough of me. But I have to go to work. So I will try to make up for it by giving her lots of attention when she wakes at night.' Although you are recognizing the cause of the problem and doing your best to meet your baby's needs, you are also sending her some confusing messages. By giving her lots of attention at night, you will reinforce her feeling that she can't manage until morning. She will also not get the idea that nighttime is for sleeping.

You have to go to work, and you would prefer your baby to

sleep all night. So what can you do? Because you have identified the cause of the waking, you can also find the solution. If you feel your baby wakes because she needs more of you, try to give her more of you – but not in the middle of the night. Perhaps you could devote your full attention to her for an hour or so before bed, so that she goes to sleep feeling loved and close to you. You might get up a bit earlier in the morning, to spend some relaxed time with your baby before you go to work. Even if what you can do doesn't seem much to you, it can feel like a great deal to your baby. Just by understanding what she is asking for, you will be able to treat her in a way that recognizes her needs, without starting a habit of waking up to see you at night.

Weaning

Weaning does not cause problems when you can follow your baby's lead, so that she starts eating solid food when she tells you she is ready and gives up the breast or bottle when she no longer needs it. If you go back to work while your baby is still breast feeding, be positive about it. Don't regret the midday feed that you can no longer share. Enjoy a close feed or two in the evening, and another in the early morning, but don't feed her in the middle of the night once she has shown she is able to sleep through (see Chapter 6). Let her go to sleep satisfied and looking forward to your reunion, refreshed and rested, in the morning.

Unwinding

When you have had a big day, try to give your baby a chance to wind down and relax before sleep. It is tempting to hurry her into bed when you come home late from a day out, but going through her routine as usual will help her settle down and give her bedtime cues.

Stick your older baby in her high chair as usual, even if all she eats is a bite of banana. Don't rush her bath. Even with a young baby you can talk over the events of the day, perhaps while looking at a picture book. It is better for her to go to bed half an hour late than to be rushed into bed while she is still hyped up with excitement and fatigue.

Formula for Coping with a Disturbed Night

Although different causes of anxiety will respond to different solutions, they are all best applied when your baby is meant to be awake, with a special focus on 'her' time during her evening routine and perhaps first thing in the morning. Babies do need a lot of attention. They respond well when they get enough and seem to protest when they don't.

The formula for handling a disturbed night is basically the same as the one for establishing good sleep patterns in the first place:

- First listen to your baby's cry. Try to decide how she is feeling. A tired cry means your baby will probably go to sleep without help. A distressed cry calls for a reassuring visit.

- Unless she sounds acutely distressed, give her a chance to go to sleep by herself. She may be half-asleep and your arrival could just wake her up fully.

- When you go to her, keep the disturbance to a minimum. Talk softly and keep the lights off or low. Pick her up only if she can't settle with patting and soothing. Don't take her out of the room. It will only confuse her more if unexpected things happen.

- Reassure her that you are there, she is loved and all is well. Remind her that it is night-time and time to go to sleep.

- Don't feed her once night feeds have been dropped. If she seems to want something, give her a drink of water.

- Repeat this drill until she is able to settle down and go to sleep.

• PROTESTS AT BEDTIME •

Bedtime protests are universal. You can be sure you will have a case of them at least once. What you can't predict is when they will show up.

Bedtime may be the moment your baby chooses to express anxiety or discomfort that has been manageable during the day.

Separating from you for the night is an especially vulnerable time for her. For this reason major bedtime protests often coincide with a developmental spurt at about nine months, when your baby is acutely aware of the possibility of separation from you.

Everything we have said about finding the cause of night-time disturbances and how to handle them also applies to bedtime protests. There is, however, one important difference.

A baby who wakes in the night isn't consciously deciding to wake herself up. In a sense, she can't help it: something is waking her, or preventing her from going back to sleep after a natural surfacing in her sleep cycle. But at about nine months your baby becomes able to prevent herself from falling asleep by using her will-power. Even if she is dropping with exhaustion, she can now refuse to go to sleep. She may use this new ability to test you to the limit. What she is really testing is whether, when you say it is bedtime, it really is bedtime; or whether she, the baby, can change the rules.

Usually the message she needs to hear is that nothing has changed. Bedtime is still bedtime, you are still in charge, and night-time is still for sleeping. There will be times, though, when you will need to make minor adjustments to keep pace with your baby's development.

———————— ★★★ ————————

UNTIL Anna was eight months old, she loved her bedtime routine with her mother and settled happily in bed. She had accomplished the move from a basket to her cot with no problems and no change in her settling routine. Her mother would tuck her in, sit down and sing a lullaby. Sometimes Anna would relax almost immediately, sometimes she would fret and toss her head a bit. But she was always ready to drop off in less than five minutes, and her mother would then say good night and leave the room.

Suddenly Anna's bedtime behaviour changed. She would kick off the covers as soon as she was put down, bounce around and sometimes shout. She ignored the lullaby she had enjoyed. Her mother started spending as long as ten minutes sitting calmly beside her cot, hoping to soothe her, but it made no difference.

When her mother left the room, Anna would cry loudly. 'What is going on?' Anna's mother asked Lucy.

'She wants you to go away,' said Lucy. 'You are creating intolerable tension for her, because she knows you are going to leave, and she can't stand waiting for you to do it. She knows how to settle herself for sleep on her own now, and she wants you to let her do it.'

So Anna's mother began singing the lullaby as she carried Anna to bed. She tucked her in, wound up a musical toy, kissed her good night and left. She was spending two minutes in the bedroom, instead of ten. Anna would give a token squawk as her mother left the room and then go to sleep.

Anna's mother found it a fascinating experience. 'I learned so much,' she said, 'about how to make definite changes as Anna grows, and how to listen to what she is telling me. I thought she needed more settling, when in fact she needed less. What was a soothing, reassuring presence for her when she was little had become infuriating, with her new awareness of what bedtime means. It reminded me that I must be prepared to drop my assumptions and always be open to new information from her.'

The thing that doesn't change is that bedtime is bedtime, whether your baby likes it or not. But how bedtime is handled can change with your baby. Behaviour like Anna's can easily be misunderstood as a refusal to go to bed, when in fact it was simply a request to change *how* she went to bed.

———— ★★★ ————

As your baby gets older, there will be genuine refusals to go to bed. If handled firmly and consistently, these will not develop into a bedtime problem. As she approaches her first birthday, your baby's world is expanding rapidly. She sees it from an exciting new perspective, as she pulls herself to standing and prepares to walk. Her mobility lets her explore everything within reach. She is on a high, completely thrilled with her discoveries, and she is also developing the strong will-power and drive to assert herself that will dominate the toddler years.

The combination can be a deadly one at bedtime. She is reluctant to give up the glories of the day and go to sleep, and she may become furious with you for insisting that she does.

My daughter developed a classic case of this at eleven months old. She would stand in her cot and yell at the top of her voice for half an hour. When I went in to settle her, her furious crying would redouble in intensity as I left. I couldn't bear the thought of her sobbing until she collapsed in an exhausted heap, but I seemed to be making it worse.

Lucy asked me to describe her behaviour. Then she said: 'She's angry that the day is over, and she's angry with you for putting her to bed. Going back in to remind her that it's bedtime just makes her crosser.'

That fitted my impression. But what could I do to help her?

'What is usually the best thing to do when someone is very angry?' asked Lucy.

'Sometimes, they need to be left alone to cool off. It really is all you can do. You've tried reassuring her and it doesn't help.'

So I had to let her go through it. I would retreat to the other end of the house and miserably do the ironing while my baby yelled. But it didn't last long. After I stopped going back in, the protests ceased within days.

If I had felt I was 'leaving her to cry', I would not have been able to do it. But Lucy reminded me that it was the proper response to my baby's needs at that stage of her development, and the fact that it was painful for me didn't mean it was painful for her. I found it distressing, but at least I didn't feel confused or guilty. My concern that my baby might feel abandoned was unfounded, as Lucy pointed out. If she had felt like that, she would have stopped crying when I went in to settle her, not cried more furiously when she realized I would not get her up again. A baby of this age has learned that you always come back, and she is unlikely, in the normal run of things, to panic about that.

Lucy suggests telling your baby that you know she is able to go to sleep by herself, without your help, and so you won't be coming back tonight and you'll see her in the morning. Or you could go in once and then tell her you won't come back again.

Your baby needs to test the boundaries of her world, so as to be able to feel secure within them. It is part of her healthy, intelligent drive to explore everything she encounters. She will probably need to test the rules about bedtime several times, at different stages of her development. She has changed, so it's only natural that she experiments to find out if the world has changed too. It is her job to test the limits, and your job to hold them in place. It can feel like quite a struggle, but giving up would only make things worse.

SLEEP PLAN FOR BAD NIGHTS

▶ Listen to your baby's cry and try to work out what she is feeling.

▶ Consider what may be causing her to wake: teething? A new stage in her development?; a change in her life, or in yours?

▶ Try to reassure her that you understand how she feels, but that it is night-time and she needs to sleep.

▶ Give your baby extra attention in the daytime if she seems to need you at night.

▶ Go back to basics. Settle your baby in the same way as you did when she was tiny and you were helping her learn to sleep.

▶ Be on the lookout for times when you may need to change your routine to suit your older baby.

▶ Remember that, as she grows, she will need regularly to test the limits that you set. She needs to feel secure boundaries around her.

9

COLIC AND OTHER PROBLEMS

'He spent six weeks in hospital after he was born, and he needed to be fed through a tube for three and a half months. When he came home, he was so jumpy and hyper-sensitive that he couldn't bear his face to be touched. Put down to sleep, he just screamed.'

Mother of Dylan, two, who now goes to bed happily and sleeps all night.

IN MOST CASES there is no physical reason why a baby shouldn't settle down and sleep through the night within the first few months of life. Indeed there is every reason why a healthy baby should. But some babies, especially ill babies, do have problems that make it more difficult for them to reach the relaxed state they need to sleep well.

It is also much harder for parents to help their baby develop healthy sleep patterns if he has been ill, or if he has a specific problem. It can feel impossible to treat him normally and to believe that he will eventually be able to sleep well. It may take him longer to get there, and he may need special kinds of help, appropriate to his particular needs. But babies with problems need their sleep just as much as, if not more than, healthy ones, so it's even more important for them that early difficulties with sleep are overcome.

If your baby has a particular medical condition, you should be given plenty of information about it, including how it may affect his ability to sleep. In this book we make no attempt to illustrate every specific problem you and your baby may face. Sleep skills are built on certain basic foundations, although the way each baby becomes master of his own sleep is unique. This method of helping babies learn to sleep is based on a number of fundamental principles, discussed in detail throughout the book. They apply to ill babies, and to babies with problems, just as they do to healthy ones. Some of them may be more difficult to remember when dealing with the extra challenges these babies present and for that very reason they are especially relevant here:

- Listen to your baby and try to work out exactly what he is feeling.

- Put your own anxieties and assumptions to one side when dealing with your baby, so as to be able to give him what he really needs, rather than what you think he ought to need.

- Send consistent messages about how the day comes to an end, and night-time is for sleep.

- Keep necessary attention at night to a minimum, and disturb your baby's night as little as possible.

- Learn to trust your baby to sleep.

Case studies prove that, when parents have the confidence to apply them, techniques for encouraging healthy babies to sleep are just as effective in helping babies with difficulties. This is true even when a baby's problems are severe, as one family's remarkable story shows.

———— ★★★ ————

DYLAN was born with no signs of life. He was resuscitated and spent nearly six weeks in hospital, first in intensive care, then in special care. He couldn't swallow, because of damage to the nerves in his mouth and throat, so he was fed through a tube for three and a half months. His inability to swallow allowed mucus to accumulate in his throat, making his breathing noisy and gurgling, and distressing to listen to.

When he finally came home from hospital, Dylan screamed nearly all the time he was awake. He could fall asleep only in his parents' arms. If they tried to put him down, he screamed. He seemed badly traumatized by his birth, and by his early days in intensive care: he couldn't bear to lie on his back, or for his face to be touched, or for clothes to be pulled over his head. By the time Dylan was three months old his mother was close to breaking point when Lucy went to see them.

Together they worked out that Dylan was comfortable only on his tummy. In this position, fluid could drain out of his mouth and he felt more secure and supported. His panic when he felt empty space around him was evidently a reaction to the extreme stress he had experienced while lying exposed on his back in the special care unit. Knowing that current advice is not to put babies face down to sleep, Lucy helped Dylan's parents experiment with different sleep positions, until they found one which gave him the sensation of pressure on his tummy that he liked. (See Chapter 7 for suggestions about sleeping positions.) Dylan started to sleep.

It was a breakthrough for the whole family. Their problems were not over, of course. Dylan still needed lots of help to settle down, and his parents had to be very clear and consistent in their handling of him, especially at night. It wasn't until he was seventeen months old that Dylan began to relax within the boundaries his parents had created, accept his bedtime and go to sleep easily. But starting to sleep was the turning point. After that Dylan coped better, and so did his parents.

Now aged two, still without a clear diagnosis of his condition, Dylan has continuing breathing and feeding difficulties, and his generally poor muscle tone means he is not yet able to walk. Despite all this he goes to sleep happily listening to music in bed and doesn't wake until morning. His mother reports that Dylan sleeps better than many of her friends' healthy children of the same age.

Dylan's parents knew he desperately needed sleep, and so did they. Their determination helped them to stick to their approach of identifying his needs and trying to meet them, while at the same time sending him clear signals about night-time being for sleep. Yet parents whose babies have much less severe problems often jump to the conclusion that there is nothing they can do to improve their baby's sleep.

--- ★★★ ---

• COLIC •

A baby who cries for no apparent reason is often said to be colicky. Typically, colic happens in the early evening, lasts for one to three hours, and disappears by the time the baby is three months old. It is thought to be linked to indigestion, because the baby will sometimes draw his knees up to his chest, as though he has stomach pain.

Your doctor may diagnose colic, and reassure you that 'he'll soon grow out of it'. A medical explanation may make it easier to cope with the daily crying spell. Certainly it helps to know it won't last forever. But there is a drawback to accepting colic as the cause of sleeplessness: the chance to use the first few months to establish good sleep habits may be missed altogether. This 'golden time', when you can take full advantage of your baby's biological readiness to adapt to sleeping all night, is soon over. On top of that, techniques used to soothe your baby when he is colicky can easily become lasting habits, making him unable to go to sleep on his own and stay asleep all night.

On the other hand, being told 'there is no such thing as colic' is not much use when you can see no reason for hours of crying every evening. There are drops available for colic; some parents find they help. If not, you may feel there is nothing you can do but wait it out. This is never true. There is always something you can do to help, or at least make a situation easier to manage, for you and for your baby. Colic is a label we use to describe a baby's behaviour. The best approach is to forget the label and consider the behaviour.

It is linked to feeding, because everything in a tiny baby is linked to feeding. Feeding is how he experiences his bodily sensations, and bodily sensations are how he experiences his emotions. Three specific feeding problems can show up as colic: underfeeding, overfeeding and confused feeding.

A baby who is underfed may manage through the day, but as evening approaches he may become ravenous and scream from hunger. However, there will usually be other signs as well, such as failing to put on weight.

Overfeeding is more likely to be the cause. A crying baby is often offered a feed in an attempt to pacify him. He may well accept a feed he doesn't want, because sucking eases his discomfort. But his overloaded digestive system will then cause renewed pain, and more screaming. A dummy, which your baby can suck without having to cope with more food, can sometimes be the answer here.

Confused feeding is very common. It happens when a baby feeds at the wrong times, when he isn't really hungry, so his body rhythms are prevented from settling into a smooth pattern. He feels dissatisfied and constantly peckish, but not hungry enough to take a proper feed, and not able to relax enough for good digestion. Again, he may get through the day, but by evening he can't cope any more and goes to pieces.

There is one theory that a new baby whose body is very tightly curled may squash his immature digestive system and cause indigestion. If you suspect this, you could try some gentle baby massage (see Chapter 7), especially after a warm bath. Tension will make your baby curl up tighter, so anything that relaxes him will help.

Occasionally colic is caused by milk intolerance, or by allergy. Neither of these applies to babies who are fed only breast milk.

Milk intolerance is when a baby can't digest his formula milk. It's usually obvious. There will be clear symptoms of digestive difficulties, such as vomiting, diarrhoea or constipation. Despite taking plenty of milk, your baby may seem underfed and fail to thrive. Crying will be linked with feeding, regardless of the time of day. Some babies cry while they feed, others afterwards. Milk intolerance sometimes shows up when a baby is weaned early from the breast. Your doctor will prescribe a different formula.

Allergy is when a baby's immune system is affected by something in his formula milk. His body becomes sensitized to it and tries to fight it off. Allergies usually show up in rashes and other skin symptoms, but they can cause stomach upsets as well. Allergies can be triggered by the complicated proteins in formula milk. Later on, when babies are eating solid food, babies who were breast fed are less likely to develop allergies. The perfect digestibility of breast milk means their systems have not been sensitized when they are very young, and they have had more time to build up their immunity.

The obvious question about colic is why it happens at the same time every day, typically between five and ten o'clock in the evening. There is an equally obvious answer. It is the end of the day. Your baby is tired, after coping with a barrage of stimuli all day long. You are tired and probably stressed. It is a busy time for this tired household: hungry people are coming home, there are meals to be cooked, other children may need attention. The intimate simplicity of your baby's day, perhaps alone with an attentive parent, is gone. He could feel fragmented, bewildered, over-stimulated and exhausted. He will be unable to feed well.

In other words, colic may be caused by stress. The answer is to give your baby lots of time to wind down in the evening. Try to avoid getting harassed yourself. Take the time to make the evening feed a close, relaxed one. Make sure that your baby isn't in an awkward position, half-turned away from you, because an uncomfortable feed will affect his digestion.

Remember, too, that your baby will absorb anxiety from you. Tensions build up when there's an audience for the baby's crying spell. Family members may put pressure on you with well-meant advice. When you are struggling with a screaming baby and someone says: 'He must be hungry', even when you're pretty sure he's not, you may offer him a feed just for the sake of a quiet life.

Don't do what other people think you should. Beyond helping to calm your baby in the ways suggested here, and in Chapter 4, ignore the colic. Carry out the programme for encouraging your baby to go to sleep, but wait until he is relaxed. If that's not until 10pm, don't worry. Keep as calm as you can, take it one day at a time and he'll settle down much sooner than he will if you become anxious or give up altogether.

Even if he goes to bed late, it's important to keep the transition between being awake and going to sleep. He can't learn good sleep habits if he drops off exhausted and wakes to find himself unexpectedly in bed. He needs to be aware of going to bed and to sleep. As your reassurance and consistent handling gradually relax him, he'll be able to go to bed earlier. For now, a calm, peaceful atmosphere is more important in helping him settle down.

• COLDS •

You will probably know your baby is ill before he has any obvious symptoms. He will just not seem his normal self. He may be pale, with dull eyes, and off his food. He may be clumsy, or less cheerful than usual. Cold symptoms often appear after a run of a few broken nights, to solve the mystery of why your baby was waking up. He was feeling rotten while he was developing a cold, just as we all do.

Again, don't change your usual night-time routine. Do what you can to help your baby cope, so that he sleeps as well as he can until he is better. He needs as much sleep as possible, to help him fight off the infection.

Babies don't get the hang of breathing through their mouths when their nose is blocked until they are two or three months old. The best way to clear a tiny baby's nose is to make him sneeze by tickling his nose with a tissue.

Being more upright will help to drain fluids that are interfering with his breathing. Put a pillow under your baby's mattress at the head end, so that he's sleeping on a slight slope. If he's very blocked up, it can help him to sleep in his car seat for a night or two. Lavender oil sprinkled on a handkerchief near his head is a gentle way to ease his breathing. You can also put a few drops in a bowl of water over a radiator.

He needs extra fluids, so offer him a drink of water if he wakes in the night. He is likely to be confused by the unpleasant new experience of having a cold, as well as uncomfortable.

Remember to reassure him that he's all right, just a bit snuffly, and he'll be able to go back to sleep soon. Don't fuss over him. Give him a chance to get back to sleep on his own for ten minutes or so before going to soothe him again. The idea is to create an atmosphere of sleep around your restless baby.

A tickly cough will give your baby disturbed nights, but it serves an important purpose in clearing fluids from his chest. Boil a kettle in his room if he has a very dry cough: the steam will ease his breathing.

You may suspect a sore throat if your baby cries when he swallows. If he touches his ear when he cries, he may have earache. Let your GP examine him in the morning.

Small babies are bad at regulating their temperature and easily get overheated. If your baby seems at all hot, take off a layer of clothing or bedding. Use natural fibres, such as cotton, which allow the skin to breathe.

• THRUSH •

Thrush is an air-borne infection. It's very common in young babies, because their immune system is underdeveloped. It will produce white plaques inside your baby's mouth and his tongue may look raw underneath. It hurts to suck, so your baby may refuse to feed, or scream while he feeds. He may seem hungry and anxious. If thrush is severe, it can go right through your baby's system and appear on his bottom as a red patch surrounded by red spots. The inflammation will make it painful for your baby to pass urine.

Thrush sometimes follows a course of antibiotics, which destroy some of the natural protective lining in the gut. It is easily treated. If you suspect thrush, see your GP.

• PREMATURE BABIES •

A baby is premature if his mother was thirty-six weeks pregnant or less when he was born. Parents are usually advised to think of their babies as the age they would have been if they had been born at full term, because the time they need to catch up with full-term babies can make them seem behind in their development.

Premature babies almost always have sleep problems, and with good reason. The pregnancy is more likely to have been difficult or stressful, and their birth is sometimes traumatic. Special care baby units are alienating, frightening places, for babies as well as for their parents.

The whole atmosphere of high-tech expertise surrounding your premature baby inevitably undermines your confidence in your own ability to care for him. Taking responsibility for him, and the everyday handling and feeding that builds communication between you, is delayed. When it does begin, it's complicated by problems stemming from your baby's early stressful experiences.

However brave and cheerful you manage to be about it, it is harrowing to have a premature baby, and, of course, to be one. It is only to be expected that high levels of anxiety colour the first few weeks at home. When you have seen your baby need help to breathe and feed, it's natural to feel you can't trust him to breathe on his own, or to let you know when he needs food. He is likely to have to be woken for feeding at first, so it's impossible for you to begin the process of letting him sleep.

In due course you have to move from this stage to learning to treat your baby as a normal, healthy infant. This can be very difficult to do. Once your doctor assures you your baby is healthy, it is a good idea to begin taking small steps towards the transition. Any demonstration of your confidence in him will help your baby make more rapid progress. If you continue to treat him as fragile and unreliable when it's no longer true, he will sense that it's not safe to sleep. The consolidation of his sleep into long stretches at night, the bone and muscle growth that goes on while he sleeps, and the hearty appetite which follows good sleep, all of which especially benefit a premature baby, will be unnecessarily delayed.

If, for example, you have been waking your baby for a feed every two hours, after you get the green light from your doctor, try letting him sleep for three hours before you wake him. If he wakes on his own and cries for food, you are on the way to learning to understand his cries, and he is on the way to discovering his needs and how to communicate them.

The anxiety that afflicts parents of a premature baby can make everything seem terribly difficult. It helps to acknowledge your own feelings, and then consciously decide to do something you know is good for your baby, rather than what you instinctively feel like doing yourself. You could call it doing what your baby needs, instead of what you want. For example, you could say to yourself 'I know I want him to wake up, because when he's awake, I'm certain he's all right. But I also know he needs good sleep. So I'm going to do what he needs, not what I want.' Then decide what time you will wake up to check on him, and go to sleep yourself.

On top of all the worry caused by what you and your baby have been through, you also have to wean him off the hospital regime, his whole experience of the world until now. If he has been accustomed to noise, disturbance and light around the clock, he may have trouble adjusting to normal rhythms of day and night. Make the distinction as clear as you can. Keep his night feeds very quiet, in the dimmest possible light – candlelight is especially peaceful. When he stops taking a really good feed when he wakes, he is ready to begin to sleep for longer stretches at night, just like a full-term baby.

• TWINS •

Twins are frequently born premature, so you have everything described above multiplied by two. When twins are born at full term, they are usually small and so likely to be extra hungry and demanding.

Some people prefer to get twins on to a strict schedule and feed them at the same time. But experience shows that it is often more successful to treat them as two separate individuals and allow them to establish their own distinct cycles of sleep and feeding. You might think this would mean you would be forever feeding. In fact one baby frequently becomes the 'team leader' and wakes for a feed first, while the other will follow soon afterwards. Once feeding is efficient, you can feed your babies one after the other in quite a short time.

The key to feeding two babies successfully is to establish a clear gap between feeds. This is important with one baby, but absolutely vital with two. If you feed two babies whenever they squawk, you will literally never stop feeding. The feeds themselves will tend to be more drawn-out, muddled affairs when your baby isn't really hungry. So parents of twins need to be extra clear that their baby is really hungry before starting a feed.

Having twins, even when you were expecting it, is a shock to the system and your confidence may be shaken at first. It seems to work better when you think of your babies as two separate people, rather than one baby multiplied by two. It means you will be able to establish clear signals with each baby right from the start and it stops you feeling quite so overwhelmed.

On top of everything else twins often sleep badly, because they wake each other up. This is all the more reason to let them find their own rhythms. One baby may mature more quickly than the other, and start sleeping through the night while his twin still needs to wake for feeds.

Colic, colds, thrush, prematurity and twins have been used here as just five examples of the kind of difficulties that can complicate the business of sleep for you and your baby, and make good sleep habits more difficult to achieve. The common thread running through these different situations, and any others you may have to deal with, is balance: while acknowledging the difficulty, and helping your baby with it, you need to believe that sleep is something he will learn to do, and to persist in conveying that belief to your baby.

SLEEP PLAN FOR ILLNESS AND DIFFICULT SITUATIONS

▶ Recognize the part played by your feelings. If you don't believe your baby can sleep well, he will find it very difficult to do so.

▶ Accept that your confidence, and your baby's, will suffer a setback. Try to send reassuring messages to your baby and to yourself.

▶ Remember that there is always something you can do to help.

▶ When your baby wakes in the night, do what is necessary and no more. Keep disturbance to a minimum. An ill baby will probably need more than a comforting pat on the back, but the principle remains the same.

▶ Adapt your sleep programme, don't abandon it. Firm guidelines are reassuring for your baby, and changes from his routine only confuse him further.

▶ Don't be misled by your baby's condition into assuming he always wakes from genuine distress. Observe him closely. A baby who wakes because he wants company and play needs quite a different response from one who is feeling ill. One needs to be told firmly that it's time for sleep. The other needs your sympathy and help.

10

GOLDEN RULES

ALTHOUGH nothing is simpler than sleep when it is going well, it's still a subtle, mysterious and complex business. It rests on a delicate balance, easily lost. Good sleep happens when you're getting a lot of things just right, whether you're aware of it or not. Because of that, uncovering the secrets of problem-free nights has led us into some varied territory.

We have seen that you need to know yourself, and your baby, quite well. It also helps to know something about the nature of sleep itself and the conditions that encourage it, as well as the close relationship between sleep and what goes in the daytime. Sleep can't be seen in isolation from your baby's emotions, habits, feeding and physical and mental development.

When we first had the idea for this book, we wanted to reveal to parents a kind of magic formula: you hold the keys that will unlock your baby's ability to sleep all night, as early, and as easily, as possible. And the approach we have described will work like magic. But when we are asked to sum it up in a sentence ('So what's the secret, then?'), we can't. Before you can apply these few, simple rules, you need to understand your baby's sleep, and the part you play in it. That's how you become the expert on your own baby's sleep.

The detail in this book is there to illuminate your baby's behaviour and help you understand it. But the true magic of this approach is its simplicity. Your baby herself will provide plenty of information as you negotiate her unexpected tricks and turns together. Individual, day-to-day variations from child to child and family to family are infinite. But the answer is always to come back to basics. The solution lies in just a handful of central principles.

In the end you will find this approach so simple and easy to use that the twelve 'golden rules' listed below will be all you need. They will work as a trouble-shooting guide, allowing you to nip sleep problems in the bud before they have a chance to grow. They are also a kind of map, to consult whenever you momentarily lose your way. Whatever is causing your baby to be wakeful, they will get you both back on track to peaceful nights.

- Never wake a healthy, sleeping baby.

- Never feed your baby at night during hours she has shown she can sleep through.

- Never let your baby go to bed holding a bottle.

- Put your baby to bed relaxed and awake.

- Let her get used to going to sleep on her own. Aim for your baby's sleep to be under her own control.

- Learn your baby's hunger cry in her earliest days and spend time developing communication with your baby, so that you can recognize her needs.

- Concentrate on identifying your baby's needs so that you can meet them appropriately. At the same time send her clear messages that night-time is for sleep and she can't change that.

- Keep contact and disturbance after bedtime to a minimum. Never play with your baby at this time, or do anything she could interpret as a reward for being awake.

- Establish a regular, enjoyable, relaxing bedtime routine from two months onwards.

- Daytime sleeps are an addition to night-time sleep, not a substitute for it.

- Recognize your own needs, feelings and attitudes and deal with them separately from your baby.

- There is always something you can do to help. Remember that doing nothing can sometimes be the right thing to do.

As your baby grows, her needs and her behaviour will change. Soon, instead of a cry in the night that needs you to interpret its meaning, you will be woken by a little person beside your bed with a story about a monster in her room, or a dream that an ostrich came to eat her. But throughout the changes in your child, the rules remain the same. Reassurance, consistency, confidence and a friendly but firm reminder that night-time is for sleeping. For everyone.

INDEX